The Kaiser Permanente Podiatry Experience: Lessons Learned in Foot and Ankle Surgery

Editor

CHRISTY M. KING

CLINICS IN PODIATRIC MEDICINE AND SURGERY

www.podiatric.theclinics.com

Consulting Editor
THOMAS J. CHANG

January 2024 • Volume 41 • Number 1

ELSEVIER

1600 John F. Kennedy Boulevard • Suite 1800 • Philadelphia, Pennsylvania, 19103-2899

http://www.theclinics.com

CLINICS IN PODIATRIC MEDICINE AND SURGERY Volume 41, Number 1
January 2024 ISSN 0891-8422, ISBN-13: 978-0-443-13061-8

Editor: Megan Ashdown
Developmental Editor: Anita Chamoli

Clinics in Podiatric Medicine and Surgery (ISSN 0891-8422) is published quarterly by Elsevier Inc., 360 Park Avenue South, New York, NY 10010-1710. Months of issue are January, April, July, and October. Business and Editorial Offices: 1600 John F. Kennedy Blvd., Ste. 1800, Philadelphia, PA 19103-2899. Customer Service Office: 3251 Riverport Lane, Maryland Heights, MO 63043. Periodicals postage paid at New York, NY and additional mailing offices. Subscription prices are $332.00 per year for US individuals, $100.00 per year for US students and residents, $417.00 per year for Canadian individuals, $505.00 for international individuals, $100.00 per year for Canadian students/residents, and $220.00 per year for foreign students/residents. For institutional access pricing please contact Customer Service via the contact information below. To receive student/resident rate, orders must be accompanied by name of affiliated institution, date of term, and the *signature* of program/residency coordinator on institution letterhead. Orders will be billed at individual rate until proof of status is received. Foreign air speed delivery is included in all *Clinics* subscription prices. All prices are subject to change without notice. POSTMASTER: Send address changes to *Clinics in Podiatric Medicine and Surgery*, Elsevier Health Sciences Division, Subscription Customer Service, 3251 Riverport Lane, Maryland Heights, MO 63043. **Customer Service: 1-800-654-2452 (US). From outside of the US, call 314-447-8871. Fax: 314-447-8029. E-mail: JournalsCustomerService-usa@elsevier.com (for print support); JournalsOnline-Support-usa@elsevier.com (for online support).**

Reprints. For copies of 100 or more of articles in this publication, please contact the Commercial Reprints Department, Elsevier Inc., 360 Park Avenue South, New York, NY 10010-1710. Tel.: 212-633-3874; Fax: 212-633-3820; E-mail: reprints@elsevier.com.

Clinics in Podiatric Medicine and Surgery is covered in *MEDLINE/PubMed (Index Medicus)* and *EMBASE/Excerpta Medica*.

Contributors

CONSULTING EDITOR

THOMAS J. CHANG, DPM
Clinical Professor and Past Chairman, Department of Podiatric Surgery, California College of Podiatric Medicine, Sonoma County Orthopedic/Podiatric Specialists, Faculty, The Podiatry Institute, Santa Rosa, California

EDITOR

CHRISTY M. KING, DPM, FACFAS, ABPM
Residency Director, Kaiser San Francisco Bay Area Foot and Ankle Residency Program, Kaiser Oakland Foundation Hospital; Attending Surgeon, Orthopedics and Podiatry Department, Foot and Ankle Surgery, Kaiser Oakland, Oakland, California

AUTHORS

FRANCESCA M. CASTELLUCCI-GARZA, DPM, FACFAS
Residency Site Director for the Diablo Service Area, Kaiser San Francisco Bay Area Foot and Ankle Residency Program, Kaiser Oakland Foundation Hospital, Oakland, California; Attending Surgeon, Orthopedics and Podiatry Department, Foot and Ankle Surgery, Kaiser Antioch, Antioch, California

DANNY J. CHOUNG, DPM
Kaiser North Bay Consortium Foot and Ankle Residency Program, Department of Orthopedics/Podiatry, Kaiser Permanente San Rafael, San Rafael, California

DAVID R. COLLMAN, DPM
Staff Surgeon, Kaiser San Francisco Bay Area Foot and Ankle Residency Program, Department of Orthopedics, Podiatry, Injury, Sports Medicine, Kaiser Permanente San Francisco Medical Center, San Francisco, California

JOSEPH D. DICKINSON, DPM
Kaiser San Francisco Bay Area Foot and Ankle Residency Program, Department of Orthopedics/Podiatry, Kaiser Permanente Oakland Medical Center, Oakland, California

SHONTAL BEHAN DIONISOPOULOS, DPM, FACFAS
The Permanente Medical Group, Diablo Service Area, Walnut Creek, California

MATTHEW B. DOBBS, MD, FACS, FAAOS, FAOA
Director of the Dobbs Clubfoot Center, Medical Director, Palm Beach International Surgery Center, Paley Institute, West Palm Beach, Florida; Senior Editor, *Clinical Orthopaedics and Related Research*; Immediate Past President, United States Bone and Joint Initiative; President-Elect, Association of Bone and Joint Surgeons; President, International Federation of Pediatric Orthopaedic Societies

LAWRENCE FORD, DPM, FACFAS
Attending Surgeon, Kaiser San Francisco Bay Area Foot and Ankle Surgery, Department of Orthopedics and Podiatric Surgery, Kaiser Permanente, Oakland, California

VARSHA SALUNKHE IVANOVA, DPM
Chief Resident, Kaiser Permanente Foot and Ankle Surgery, Santa Clara, California

CHRISTY M. KING, DPM, FACFAS, ABPM
Residency Director, Kaiser San Francisco Bay Area Foot and Ankle Residency Program, Kaiser Oakland Foundation Hospital; Attending Surgeon, Orthopedics and Podiatry Department, Foot and Ankle Surgery, Kaiser Oakland, Oakland, California

CRAIG E. KRCAL Jr, DPM
Fellow, The CORE Institute, Phoenix, Arizona; Kaiser San Francisco Bay Area Foot and Ankle Residency Program Alumni Class of 2023

JESSICA LICKISS, DPM, FACFAS
Site Director, Orthopedics Department, Kaiser Permanente Santa Clara Residency Program, Kaiser Permanente GSAA, San Leandro, California

LUKE J. MCCANN, DPM, FACFAS, PT
Kaiser South San Francisco Medical Center, South San Francisco, California

CRISTIAN NEAGU, DPM
Program Director, Kaiser Permanente Santa Clara Foot and Ankle Surgery, Santa Clara, California

SANDEEP PATEL, DPM, FACFAS
Attending Staff, San Francisco Bay Area Foot and Ankle Residency, Chief of Podiatry, The Permanente Medical Group, Diablo Service Area, Walnut Creek, California

JASON D. POLLARD, DPM, FACFAS
Attending Staff, Department of Orthopaedics and Podiatry, Kaiser San Francisco Bay Area Foot and Ankle Residency Program, Kaiser Foundation Hospital, Oakland, California

LINDSAY H. RUSSEL, DPM
Department of Orthopedics, Kaiser Permanente South Sacramento Medical Center, Sacramento, California

MONTE JAY SCHMALHAUS, DPM
Arlington Heights, Illinois

JOHN M. SCHUBERTH, DPM
Foot and Ankle Surgeon, of Orthopaedic Surgery, Foot and Ankle Surgery, Kaiser Permanente Medical Center, Kaiser Foundation Hospital, San Francisco, California

KHANH PHUONG SIEU TONG, DPM, MSc
Resident, Kaiser Permanente Foot and Ankle Surgery, Santa Clara, California

STEPHEN SILVANI, DPM
Diplomate and Past President, American Board of Foot and Ankle Surgeons; Fellow, American College of Foot and Ankle Surgery, Past President, American College of Foot and Ankle Pediatrics, Advisor, International Foot and Ankle Foundation, Attending Staff Emeritus, The Kaiser San Francisco Bay Area Foot and Ankle Residency Program

GLENN WEINRAUB, DPM, FACFAS
Past President, Orthopedics Department, American College of Foot and Ankle Surgery, Kaiser Permanente Santa Clara Residency Program, Kaiser Permanente GSAA, San Leandro, California

GRAY WILLIAMS, DPM, FACFAS
Podiatric Surgery Residency Director, Kaiser Permanente Foot and Ankle Surgery, Vallejo, California

MITZI L. WILLIAMS, DPM, FACFAS, FACFAP
Professor and Attending Surgeon, Director of Pediatric Foot and Ankle Deformity Clinic, Kaiser San Francisco Bay Area Foot and Ankle Residency Program, Department of Orthopedics and Podiatric Surgery, Kaiser Permanente, Oakland, California

Contents

Traditionally, the Kite manipulation and casting were utilized for the treatment of the congenital clubfoot. This was followed by an extensive posterior medial soft tissue surgical release followed by more casting. Often, the results were less than optimal with scarred, painful feet that needed further corrective surgery. Dr. Ponseti developed a different technique of manipulation, casting, and an Achilles tenotomy that fully corrected these clubfeet without the need for the extensive surgery. This was followed by the mandatory use of night braces with special shoes for a period of 4 years. The Ponseti method is now universally utilized around the world and is the standard of care for the management of clubfoot. I was fortunate to have been personally trained by Dr. Ponseti, and I have exclusively practiced this technique for the past 25 years.

The Ponseti method has proven to be successful in the treatment of both isolated and non-isolated clubfoot. The method should be executed prior to any pediatric invasive procedures and likewise should be attempted with any pediatric recurrence. A thorough neurologic examination and attention to clinical signs will help distinguish the atypical clubfoot. Despite this approach some children do require return to serial casting, physical therapy, and or surgery to achieve a plantigrade functional foot. Bracing strategies at a time of growth remain key.

Understanding the evolution of the human foot from a flexible grasping structure to one that is designed for upright posture and locomotion is paramount to treating patients with foot pain and dysfunction. Almost 100 years ago, Dudley Morton observed that certain retained atavistic traits are responsible for pathologic breakdown of the modern foot. Cadaveric research under the direction of Jeffrey Christensen provided evidence that lengthening the gastrocnemius and stabilizing the medial column helped correct the faulty biomechanics associated with Morton foot and corroborated Hansen's blueprint for reconstructive surgery of the foot and ankle.

Hallux valgus is a common foot deformity in which many surgical techniques have been introduced. Originally, Paul Lapidus detailed a midfoot arthrodesis technique to address the deformity and medial column instability that served as the foundation for the modified Lapidus bunionectomy. The appreciation of the multiplanar nature of hallux valgus deformity continues to evolve and helps to guide the investigation of the ideal surgical correction to yield more predictable results and reduced complications. Various fixation constructs have been used over the years for the Lapidus bunionectomy without a clear superior fixation technique, and literature supports early weight-bearing with each.

The traditional postoperative management of common foot and ankle procedures has involved a prolonged period of immobilization and nonweight bearing. The concern was loss of correction and fixation failure. However, it has been shown that a prolonged period of nonweight bearing can predispose patients possible deep vein thrombosis, disuse osteopenia, cardiovascular complications, and generalized deconditioning. The authors' institution has published studies reviewing the efficacy of early weight bearing after first metatarsophalangeal joint arthrodesis, modified Lapidus bunionectomy, and open reduction and internal fixation of ankle fractures. This article highlights the literature and rationale supporting the safety of early weight-bearing protocols.

Successful outcomes in the surgical treatment of the fractured ankle require methods that respect the soft tissue envelope and establish a stable mortise for functional rehabilitation. Ankle fractures in patients with osteopenia and in diabetic patients with deranged bone remodeling constitute high-risk injuries that may result in catastrophic complications. These patients present unique care challenges and should not be approached in the same manner as their healthy counterparts. We present the principles of treatment in high-risk ankle fractures, operative treatment philosophy illustrating techniques frequently used at our institution, and a review of current literature.

Foot and ankle surgeons are commonly confronted with the surgical dilemma on when and how to best surgically address trimalleolar ankle fractures with a posterior malleolar component. This may involve either direct fixation of the posterior malleolus or indirect stabilization with the fixation of the medial and lateral malleoli and trans-syndesmotic fixation. Recently there has been a paradigm shift in the management of these injuries with a more thorough understanding of anatomy, stability, and long-term sequela of these injuries. This article aims to evaluate the current literature on posterior malleolar ankle fractures, approaches to fixing the posterior malleolus, and outcomes and complications of these procedures.

In recent years, total ankle replacement (TAR) has gained widespread acceptance as a surgical treatment for end-stage ankle arthritis. This shift is due to notable improvements in implant design, surgical instrumentation, technique, and surgeon expertise, resulting in high levels of patient satisfaction comparable to ankle fusion. Additionally, indications for TAR have expanded to include advanced deformities that were previously considered unsuitable for the procedure, making ankle arthrodesis the only option. Despite these advancements, TAR still carries a higher complication rate compared to other ankle surgeries. The complex anatomy of the ankle, coupled with limited soft tissue, presents significant challenges in managing complications associated with TAR.

Charcot deformity is a challenging condition often leading to foot and ankle deformity that subsequently causes decreased function, ulceration, infection, and limb loss. There are various treatment measures to take into consideration when managing these patients. Treatment approaches range from conservative casting to surgical reconstruction. The authors believe that when faced with deformity, aggressive reconstruction to maintain a plantigrade foot and prevent loss of function is critical. Because of the nature of the Charcot condition, timing and fixation are often debated. This article discusses the authors' approach to Charcot reconstruction in a large integrated health care system.

The Achilles tendon has a high incidence of ruptures often occurring in weekend warriors and the aging population. Based on anatomic studies of the Achilles tendon, ruptures are commonly found in the watershed area proximal to the insertion site. Traditionally, treatment options included conservative therapy with immobilization and a prolonged non-weight-bearing phase versus surgical treatment. Surgical treatment can vary between open, minimally invasive, or percutaneous approaches. In more recent years, early functional rehabilitation with or without surgery has shown to have successful results.

Surgical complications are a part of every surgeon's practice. Managing your own complications or one from another provider requires carefully reviewing your patient's previous experience and surgery along with balancing their expectations. In order to provide the best treatment plan, a thorough analysis of the pre and postoperative period that contributed to the patient's outcome must be considered. Identifying what revision options are available and weighing the potential future complications that could arise from another surgery must be reviewed. Honest conversations regarding revision options and if revision surgery is even a viable option is vital for a good patient-physician relationship and outcome.

Podiatric residency is only three years to gather as many experiences to understand the various aspects of foot and ankle care including, surgery, clinics, academics, and research to prepare them for the rest of their career. It is also important to find a supportive environment to maximize both education and wellness during these naturally challenging times. The three separate Kaiser Northern California Podiatric Residency Programs have worked diligently to provide a comprehensive opportunities and experiences in all aspects of podiatric resident education.

In this article I reflect on almost 40 years of clinical practice. I remember the first day like it was yesterday, and I remember the last day, but the in between represents my soul, a soul that has been shaped by countless experiences. Some of these experiences were immediately impactful and left an indelible mark on my soul, but most of them were memorable only for a fleeting moment, soon to be forgotten. Yet the cumulation of these seemingly trivial experiences, in retrospect, served as the foundation of my career at Kaiser Permanente.

CLINICS IN PODIATRIC
MEDICINE AND SURGERY

SERIES OF RELATED INTEREST

Orthopedic Clinics
https://www.orthopedic.theclinics.com/
Clinics in Sports Medicine
https://www.sportsmed.theclinics.com/
Foot and Ankle Clinics
https://www.foot.theclinics.com/
Physical Medicine and Rehabilitation Clinics
https://www.pmr.theclinics.com/

THE CLINICS ARE AVAILABLE ONLINE!
Access your subscription at:
www.theclinics.com

Foreword

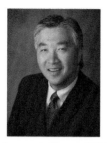

Thomas J. Chang, DPM
Consulting Editor

I have always been drawn to and inspired by educational institutions within our profession.

The schools of Podiatric Medicine deserve our gratitude and appreciation for their unwavering dedication to educating our students. For our graduates, the American College of Foot and Ankle Surgeons (ACFAS), the American Podiatric Medical Association (APMA), The Podiatry Institute (PI), and the International Foot and Ankle Foundation (IFAF) have been consistent for over 30 years in providing a consistent product for CMEs to stay current with the state-of-the-art.

Throughout my career, there have been several organizations that have impressed me as a source of tremendous quality and innovation. One of the most impressive by far is the Kaiser Permanante–Northern California group. As a student, I was exposed to the teachings of Drs Steve DeValentine, Barry Scurran, John Steinstra, Jack Schuberth, Steve Silvani, and Flair Goldman, just to name a few. They were each tremendous educators, recognized authors, and skilled surgeons, who combined to bring a level of excellence to our profession and earned parity among their orthopedic colleagues. Since these early years, their quality has been maintained by following along in the tradition of hiring the highest quality of physicians to secure their legacy. This impressive list of Northern California Kaiser physicians from the early 1980's and onward reads like a list of "Who's Who" in our field of Podiatric Medicine and Surgery.

I wanted to highlight this remarkable group of podiatric physicians as setting a standard in education, research, and surgery. Their commitment to quality is clear and something we can all aspire to. I am grateful to Dr Christy King for her efforts in bringing

Clin Podiatr Med Surg 41 (2024) xiii–xiv
https://doi.org/10.1016/j.cpm.2023.09.003
0891-8422/24/© 2023 Published by Elsevier Inc.

this issue to us. You will see a wonderful collection of many familiar and new names, and I hope you enjoy more insights and experiences from this special group of doctors.

Thomas J. Chang, DPM
Sonoma County Orthopedic/Podiatric Specialists
3536 Mendocino Avenue, Suite 300B
Santa Rosa, CA 95403, USA

E-mail address:
thomaschang14@comcast.net

Preface

Standing on the Shoulders of Giants: Podiatry's Turbulent Climb to the Pinnacle at the Northern California Kaiser Permanente Health Care System

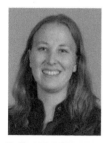

Christy M. King, DPM
Editor

(Inspired by interviews [in alphabetical order] from Drs Breivis, Fagan, Ford, Kiest, Schuberth, Scurran, and Silvani.)

When we are fortunate enough to practice within a system that allows us to treat patients effectively and efficiently at the top of our scope of practice, it is necessary to appreciate the foundation that was built by our predecessors. It is directly because of their dedication and efforts that we secured our harmonious partnership within Kaiser Permanente Northern California (KPNC). Ever since its humble beginnings, Kaiser Permanente was a revolutionary idea that strove to provide the best care for its patients with an efficient, physician-driven, and cost-conscious system. The concept of Kaiser Permanente revolves around a combination of three complementary systems: including a private insurance company, a not-for-profit hospital system, and one of the largest physician groups in the country, known as The Permanente Medical Group (TPMG). These entities have an exclusive contract with one another to work together to provide care for their patients. Outside of our walls, podiatrists compete with orthopedic physicians in the fee-for-service models for business; however, within the walls of KPNC, we partner together to deliver the highest quality of care for the patients with a cost-effective model. But, you may ask, how did we get here?

Clin Podiatr Med Surg 41 (2024) xv–xviii
https://doi.org/10.1016/j.cpm.2023.05.001
0891-8422/24/© 2023 Published by Elsevier Inc.

podiatric.theclinics.com

GETTING A SEAT AT THE TABLE (WITHOUT RESERVATIONS)

Prior to the 1970s, podiatrists were known primarily for the care of the forefoot. During the mid-1970s, opportunities presented where hospital leaders and care providers were looking for qualified podiatric practitioners in the community to join Kaiser Permanent to help manage the large backlog of patients requiring expert care of the foot and ankle. Some of the earliest hires included Drs James Larose in Kaiser Vallejo (1973), Ron Uhlman in Kaiser Vallejo (1973), and Barry Scurran at Kaiser Hayward (1974). In the early years at Kaiser Hayward, the podiatrists were hired by the innovative general surgery department to help them with diabetic foot and ankle care. Throughout the integration of podiatrists into the Kaiser Permanente system, the individual hospital locations and departments continuously monitored its practitioners to ensure the level of care provided by its podiatrists was meeting all standards. In addition to building their own podiatry departments, the podiatrists at the Kaiser Hayward and Vallejo were among the earliest sites to start podiatry residency programs on the West Coast. From the beginning, Kaiser Permanente podiatry practiced diligence, excellence in a high level of patient care, and commitment to the education of the next generation of podiatrists.

Whispers of the talent and persistence of the first Kaiser Permanente podiatrists started to spread around the San Francisco Bay Area. It was the forward thinking of Kaiser San Francisco Orthopedic Chief and Mayo Clinic–trained, Dr Jim Breivis, who developed the concept of Regional Chiefs Meetings across the Northern California area, where the early experiences with podiatrists providing quality care were further shared. This allowed more sites to experiment with this once-foreign idea. Some of the earliest podiatrists were sent to work at various Bay Area locations to promote the benefit of foot and ankle care provided by podiatric clinicians and surgeons. When asked about some of the challenges during the earlier years, Dr Scurran notes, "There is no impossible. Sometimes it just may take a little more time or monetary support." The diligent work of Dr Scurran could not be denied, and he was asked to take on increasing responsibilities and positions, including Physician-In-Chief (2005–2011) and Chief Compliance Officer. Now that there was a seat at the table for podiatry, further advancements could be made.

EXPANDING SKILL SETS WITHIN KAISER PERMANENTE NORTHERN CALIFORNIA

The next step in this revolutionary concept came when Kaiser San Francisco Orthopedic Chief, Dr Breivis, hired podiatric surgeon, Dr Jack Schuberth, and orthopedic surgeon, Dr Curt Kiest, in 1984. Dr Schuberth is a dedicated, Chicago-deep-dish-loving podiatric surgeon who completed his residency training with the Harborview group in Seattle, Washington and the talented, understanding orthopedic surgeon, Dr Sig Hansen. Dr Curt Kiest is an incredibly intelligent, open-minded orthopedic surgeon who attended Harvard and then Columbia Medical School, and then completed his residency at UCSF. It was during his time on residency rotations at UCSF that he built a friendship with a fellow resident who just happened to be a podiatrist, and she opened his eyes to all that doctors of podiatric medicine can do. Traditionally, a patient with a severe diabetic wound would mainly be provided with one option, which was a below-the-knee amputation. However, Drs Schuberth and Kiest saw an opportunity for salvaging these limbs and taking these sick patients off the hands of the general surgeons assigned on call that day. They developed a strong partnership and worked together tirelessly to take care of the Kaiser Permanente patients in the San Francisco Bay Area for decades. Relationships like this were being established at different locations around the San Francisco Bay Area, allowing podiatry to further evolve its position within KPNC. In his time in San Francisco, Dr Schuberth was the first podiatric surgeon to perform ankle open reduction internal fixations (ORIFs) and other complicated rearfoot and ankle procedures under the surveillance of his orthopedic chief, opening the door for expanding the skill sets performed by KPNC podiatric surgeons. Ultimately, he was able to expand his work to total ankle arthroplasty with the support of the orthopedic chief and department. All across the San Francisco Bay Area, KPNC Podiatry was able to start to broaden their expertise from the forefoot into the rearfoot and ankle as well.

FIGHTING FOR PARITY AND PARTNERSHIP

It took almost twenty-five years from the original podiatric hires and many tireless hours of hard-working quality care for the next big step, which involved gaining further parity as the podiatrists obtained TPMG partnership in 1998. In the 1990s, with the support of a plastic surgeon turned TPMG executive director named Dr Robert Pearl, KPNC podiatrists earned partnership within TPMG. Among all caregivers for the foot and ankle, this consistent level of parity across an organization between physicians and podiatric clinicians and surgeons is not often observed reliably around the country. As partners, podiatrists could take high leadership positions, such as Dr Scurran becoming Physician-In-Chief of Hayward (2005–2011) and then Regional Chief Compliance Officer.

OPENING DOORS AND LEAVING THEM OPEN FOR THE FUTURE GENERATIONS

Following the early collegial work of Kaiser Permanente podiatrists and orthopedic physicians as well as the supportive system of KPNC, podiatry not only found a home but also excelled in the care of the foot and ankle. In the current atmosphere, there are over 120 podiatrists working alongside 9500 Kaiser Permanente physicians, taking care of over 4 million members in the San Francisco Bay Area. At the Kaiser Northern California locations, most if not all the foot and ankle care is provided by these talented podiatric surgeons and clinicians. Along with all departments within Kaiser Permanente, quality of care is constantly reviewed, and the various podiatry providers and departments are consistently performing well. The excellent work of KPNC podiatrists helped them earn high-level positions, such as Physician-In-Chief and Assistant Physician-In-Chief, and one podiatrist is the Chief of their orthopedic department. To further strengthen relationships, podiatry residents are educated and work alongside residents in multiple medical fields, including general surgery, obstetrics and gynecology, internal medicine, head and neck surgery, psychiatry, and orthopedics. At some facilities, podiatry residents take primary orthopedic calls, which further solidifies relationships with other specialty departments. TPMG attending podiatrists and residents have produced hundreds of research articles, publications, book chapters, and presentations, which have contributed to knowledge and advancement within the profession.

The parity and respect for podiatrists within our system are unmatched as a whole across the country, allowing TPMG podiatrists to take great care of its patients' foot and ankle ailments while also affording the benefits of partnership and collaboration. We are thankful to the early arduous work and diligence of our predecessors along with the opportunities provided by our colleagues and system. A solid foundation has been constructed by our forerunners, and it is our duty to continue to build upon their revolutionary work. It is essential that we continue to provide literature-supported, cost-conscious, high-quality patient care and help to advance our profession within this supportive system. As we further shape Kaiser Permanente podiatry, it is important to keep the door open for the next generation to take our profession even further.

There are so many to thank for their early persistence and dedication, and we would like to thank the following individuals (in alphabetical order):

Jim Breivis, MD	James O. Johnston, MD	Barry Scurran, DPM
Steve DeValentine, DPM	Jeff Karlin, DPM	Larry Sheridan, DPM
Jim Fagan, DPM	Curt Kiest, MD	Stephen Silvani, DPM
Lawrence Ford, DPM	Robert Pearl, MD	Gordon Sinclair, DPM
Flair Goldman, DPM	Shannon Rush, DPM	John Steinstra, DPM
Graham Hamilton, DPM	Jack Schuberth, DPM	Ron Ulhman, DPM

Christy M. King, DPM
Kaiser Oakland Foundation Hospital
Foot & Ankle Surgery
Orthopedics and Podiatry Department
Kaiser Oakland
275 MacArthur Boulevard, Clinic 17
Oakland, CA 94611, USA

E-mail address:
Christy.m.king@kp.org

The Evolution of the Treatment of Clubfoot from Posterior Medial Release to the Ponseti Technique

My 42-Year Journey at the Permanente Medical Group

Stephen Silvani, DPM[a,b,c,d,e,*]

KEYWORDS

- Clubfoot casting • Clubfoot surgery • Ponseti • Pediatric deformity

KEY POINTS

- The Kite method of manipulation was historically used to treat clubfeet. After a period of casting, an extensive posterior medial soft tissue surgical release was performed to help correct the deformity.
- Dr Ponseti pioneered a method of manipulation and a percutaneous Achilles tenotomy that effectively corrected these clubfeet without the extensive surgery.
- The Ponseti method has been universally accepted globally and is the standard of care for the treatment of clubfeet.

INTRODUCTION: HOW IT ALL STARTED

Just before I graduated college, I was fortuitously made aware of the existence of podiatry. I liked what I found when I further investigated this field and never regretted my choice of the profession of podiatric medicine and surgery. I entered the California College of Podiatric Medicine in San Francisco in 1974.

We had courses in "podopediatrics" during my studies in podiatry school. These mostly involved lower extremity growth and development, biomechanics, metatarsus adductus, the treatment of intoed gait, and warts. Clubfoot was briefly mentioned as a severe congenital deformity with complicated surgical repairs that produced less than

[a] American Board of Foot and Ankle Surgeons; [b] American College of Foot and Ankle Surgery; [c] American College of Foot and Ankle Pediatrics; [d] International Foot and Ankle Foundation; [e] The Kaiser San Francisco Bay Area Foot and Ankle Residency Program
* c/o Christy King, DPM, Podiatric Surgery Department, 3600 Broadway, Oakland, CA 94611.
E-mail address: silvanistephen@gmail.com

Clin Podiatr Med Surg 41 (2024) 1–16
https://doi.org/10.1016/j.cpm.2023.06.001
0891-8422/24/© 2023 Elsevier Inc. All rights reserved.

satisfactory results in the long term (**Figs. 1** and **2**). I was impressed that these patients could have problems with their feet for their lifetime despite timely initial treatment.

I was a voracious reader and purchased many textbooks in school. I never like the diluted and sometimes erroneous class notes and preferred reading the authors' ideas in books and perusing the illustrations. One of my many favorites was the classic by J. H. Kite "The Clubfoot" published in 1964.[1] I read it cover to cover and studied the manipulation and casting instructions intently, but wasn't too sure about forcing correction by wedging the cast containing a supple infant foot (**Fig. 3**). Yet, I was fascinated by the ability of turning a severe congenital, crippling foot deformity into a life-transforming correction.

During my junior year of podiatry school, Dr. Ronald Uhlman, DPM came to speak to our class about his externship and residency program at the Kaiser Foundation Hospital at Vallejo, California. I was intrigued by the fact that podiatrists were respected and fully integrated into a multispecialty medical group and were highly surgical. They practiced full scope and treated infants and children. At the time mainstream medicine had yet to fully embrace "systemized" medicine and the pre-paid, non-fee-for service model. Actually, all Kaiser physicians were scorned and considered second class by the medical societies at that time. I still had no idea that my future would be a 42-year-long career at The Permanente Medical Group (TPMG).

IGNITING MY PASSION

I was fortunate to be accepted into a second-year podiatric surgical residency at The Permanente Medical Group in Hayward, California in 1978. My mentors were Barry Scurran, DPM, Jeffrey Karlin, DPM and Steven DeValentine, DPM. Immediately, I was immersed in intense, full scope, cradle-to-grave patient treatment, including exposure to the management of clubfeet. We would be called to the nursery or neonatal unit immediately after an infant was born to evaluate its clubfeet. A thorough examination was performed to rule out any other congenital issues (**Fig. 4**). DDH or spine problems were referred to pediatric orthopedics, neuromuscular concerns to pediatric neurology, and syndromic involvement was sent to genetics. The manipulation, casting and surgical repair of the feet was left entirely in our domain. This was truly a seamless, multispecialty approach to these potentially complex patients, and I enjoyed being part of

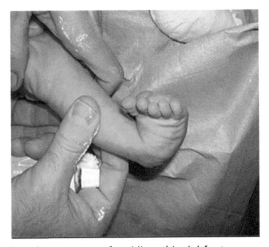

Fig. 1. The typical clinical appearance of an idiopathic clubfoot.

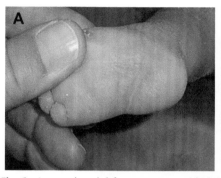
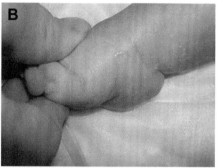

Fig. 2. A complex clubfoot presents with (*A*) a deep plantar crease and (*B*) rigid equinus with a deep posterior crease, severe plantarflexion of the metatarsals, and a short, hyperextended hallux. This less common presentation requires modification of the typical technique.[28]

the team. Relieving the parents' anxiety, managing the pedal deformity, and watching the patients grow, adapt, and flourish was very gratifying.

Consistent with the standard of practice and accepted customary procedure of the time, a modified Kite manipulation was performed. This was followed by weekly serial casting for a period of time until the eventual extensive posterior medial surgical release was necessary, usually around 1 year of age. Casting and serial manipulations rarely fully corrected these feet. Basically, the deformities were maintained until the infant was old enough to undergo general anesthesia. Through various skin incisions (most commonly the extensile posterior-medial approach as described by Turco), all soft tissue contractures were released. The shortened tendons were lengthened and repaired, the bones and joints were realigned and held with k-wires in the corrected position[2] (**Fig. 5**). Difficult to position and hard to interpret intra-operative radiographs were obtained. Casts were applied for 6 to 8 weeks to allow the corrected foot

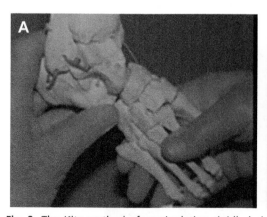
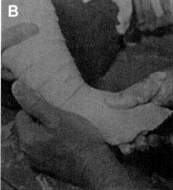

Fig. 3. The Kite method of manipulation rigidly held the calcaneus while abducting the forefoot. This would not allow the calcaneus to swing out from underneath the talus and couldn't correct the deformity. (*A*) The thumb/hand was placed over the calcaneal cuboid joint for counter pressure while the forefoot was being abducted in the traditional Kite method of manipulation. (*B*) This prevented the calcaneus from everting out from underneath the talus, effectively preventing reduction of the deformity.

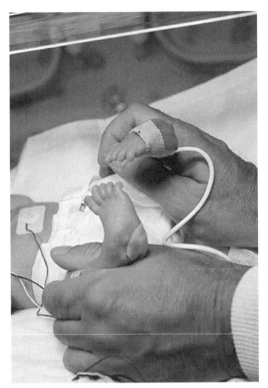

Fig. 4. The examination of the hips to rule out DDH in a premature infant with bilateral clubfeet is performed in the isolette incubator.

to heal, and then the vigorous range of motion was initiated. Maintenance was achieved via braces, therapeutic shoes, AFOs and night splints, often followed with pediatric physical therapy. Some patients would need further surgery via various salvage procedures.

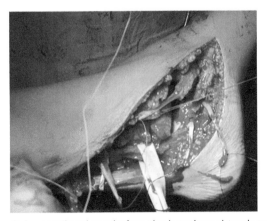

Fig. 5. A typical medial extensile release before the lengthened tendons are repaired. The drain is placed around the neurovascular bundle to mobilize and protect it during dissection.

Initially, we operated with the patients in the supine position, which made the medial work easier with the good visualization of the talonavicular release and repositioning. However, this made the posterior Achilles lengthening, the ankle and subtalar joint releases, and any lateral investigation extremely difficult. Later due to favorable reports in the literature and seminar discussions by experts in the field, we adopted starting the procedure with the patient prone, which greatly facilitated performing the posterior release (**Fig. 6**). This also helped to avoid entering the distal tibial epiphysis, which could be easily mistaken for the ankle joint, particularly in feet with severe equinus and an anteriorly positioned talus along with a thin wedged shaped posterior body. The patient was then flipped, either sterilely or with re-prepping to complete the medial release which was then easily visualized. It remained difficult to obtain proper orthogonal intra-operative radiographs that were often suboptimal, making it hard to interpret the position of the wires, completeness of the release, or adequacy of correction.

If the clubfoot was bilateral, a double-team approach was utilized. There would be 2 complete surgical teams and set-ups, including 2 surgeons, 2 residents, 2 scrub technicians, dual mayo stands, and so forth. Arm boards were utilized at the foot of the table to spread the legs, allowing the teams to efficiently work around each other.

During the 80's and early 90's, we continued to modify and perfect our approaches and procedures over numerous cases. It was typical to have all components of the deformity visualized, released, and correction achieved before letting down the tourniquet at about 1 hour. However, inserting the k-wires, reapproximating the tendons, skin closure, dressing, and casting took more time. Skin incision closure was often difficult as it was performed under tension, and wound healing was always a concern.

INCREASING UNDERSTANDING OF THE COMPLEX DEFORMITY

I continued to add to my clubfoot knowledge and understanding while perfecting my surgical technique by attending many seminars where pediatric orthopedic experts discussed the difficulty of clubfoot repair and the non-predictable outcomes. Relapses, recurrence, over and under correction were frequently reported, and revision surgeries were discussed and argued over. Long-term results of these extensive releases were increasingly being reported as less than satisfactory.

In the early 1980's I listened to Alvin Crawford, MD from Cincinnati Children's Hospital report on a novel posterior transverse fishmouth incisional approach at the Tachdjian's Pediatric Orthopedic International Seminar. This incision provided excellent access to all aspects of the deformity and was readily adopted by the clubfoot surgical community.[3] I was enthusiastic initially, but soon found in many cases it

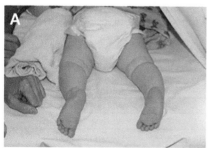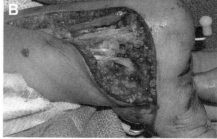

Fig. 6. The prone positioning is demonstrated in this case. (*A*) The prone surgical position is shown here. (*B*) The pin holds to correction of the subtalar joint

was very difficult to close the skin particularly in those feet with severe posterior contractures. Sometimes, the foot was left in equinus casting post-operatively for 2 or 3 weeks to allow for skin healing. Then the patient was returned to the OR for a quick cast change with the foot properly dorsiflexed, after the skin healed. It was found that although this approach facilitated the ease of surgery, it violated some of the foot angiosomes leading to wound complications and was abandoned in favor of the Turco approach.

During this time, I read with interest many journal articles on the continuing clubfoot debates about etiology, best treatment, casting techniques, surgical procedures, revisions, and outcome reviews for this challenging deformity. I continued to add to my clubfoot textbook library while trying to fully understand this complex deformity (**Table 1**).

It was obvious from the literature and my experience that clubfoot treatment outcomes were not always predictable and a poorer prognosis becomes apparent years later. In relatively short-term follow-up (2–8 years) studies, 52% to 91% good or excellent results are reported. The results rapidly deteriorate, however, as seen in longer term follow-up reports (10–25 years).[8–10] These feet can be painful, stiff, scarred, weakened, arthritic, and many have undergone multiple subsequent operations. Avascular necrosis and flat top talus, as well as other rearfoot anatomic disruptions were seen after the soft tissue release[10,11] (**Fig. 7**). Complications caused by vascular embarrassment include wound slough, infections, ischemic necrosis and limb loss.[12,13] Overcorrection with heel valgus, pes plano valgus, calcaneus deformity as well as loss of surgical correction with residual equinus, heel varus, and forefoot adductus were commonly seen.[2,14,15] Pes cavus and dorsal bunion are persistent. Limb length discrepancies have been reported, especially in unilateral deformities.[16]

By the 1990's, clubfoot surgery was being performed at multiple Permanente Medical Group facilities throughout the Northern California region. These practitioners would routinely discuss their procedures and outcomes at our quarterly conferences. Best practices were developed, technique tips shared and frustrating outcomes analyzed. This was documented in a article reviewing the Kaiser clubfoot experience from 1980 to 1990, by Blakeslee and DeValentine.[17] They reported 46% excellent, 24% good, fair 13%, and 17% poor/failures in the average follow-up of 67.2 months. These findings paralleled and confirmed the many results discussed in lectures and reported in peer-reviewed studies published at the time, as well as my own experience (**Fig. 8**).

THE BAJA PROJECT FOR CRIPPLED CHILDREN

Early in these decades, The Baja Project for Crippled Children was formed by a group of Southern Californian podiatrists (a former classmate, several upperclassmen, and

Table 1		
Clubfoot textbooks as acquired chronologically		
Year of Publication	**Title**	**Author**
1981	The Clubfoot[4]	Wallace Lehman, MD
1982	Clubfoot[5]	Vincent Turco, MD
1992	Foot and Ankle Disorders in Children[6]	Steven DeValentine, DPM
1994	The Clubfoot: The Present and a View of the Future[7]	George Simons, MD

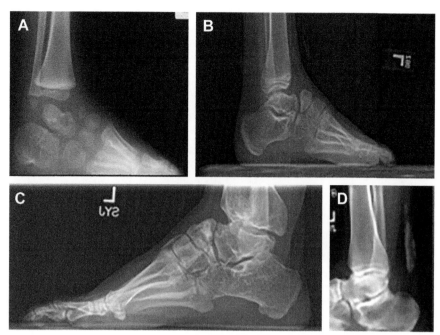

Fig. 7. Typical radiographic results are short and long term after the extensive posterior medial soft tissue surgical release. (*A*) Residual equinus and a dorsally displaced navicular are seen in this short term result. Note the posteriorly displaced fibular due to the technique of rigidly holding the rearfoot and externally rotating the foot. (*B*) This ossifying navicular is wedged shaped and dorsally located. Note the residual cavus not fully corrected by this technique. (*C*) A flat topped talus with early degenerative changes and plantarflexed first ray are seen in this older patient postoperatively. (*D*) Severe tibiotalar arthritic changes and calcification of the repaired Achilles tendon are demonstrated in this adult foot.

others) who had an interest and developed an expertise in clubfoot repair and provided treatment to underserved and neglected pediatric patients south of the border. They initially treated patients at a clinic in Mexicali, then expanded to Tijuana, Mexico in the 1980's. During the 1990's, they went to San Miguel, El Salvador, where they continued helping numerous children with neglected clubfeet as well as other congenital deformities and neuromuscular disorders. In the early 2000's, an annual weeklong surgical mission to the Hospital San Felipe in Tegucigalpa, Honduras was initiated and continues presently. An incredible number of patients received appropriate care and their lives were changed for the better by this group of dedicated physicians.

These severely crooked feet which were upside down and facing backwards defied simple releases in teenaged patients (**Fig. 9**). Commonly, a talectomy and large lateral column wedge resection were necessary to get these feet plantigrade and quasi functional. Follow-up care was provided by the local orthopedists and the patients were seen on a yearly basis on the next mission. Lectures and demonstrations were presented to the Honduran physician community, residents, and nurses on how the recognize and treat clubfeet to prevent these deformities from being neglected.

To fund raise for their mission trips abroad, The Baja Project held an annual seminar in Los Angeles with an emphasis on discussing the treatment of clubfoot from simple releases to their complicated repairs. Here again the long-term results presented were

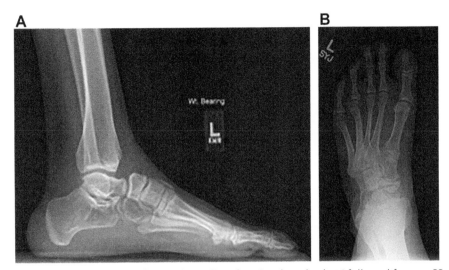

Fig. 8. This is a surgical clubfoot with excellent functional results that I followed for over 32 years. He played college football, drove a stick car and functioned at a high level with minimal symptoms. (*A*) These radiographs demonstrate well reduced equinus, an elevated navicular and a flat topped talus. (*B*) There is early degenerative changes of the talo-navicular joint with overall satisfactory alignment.

less than ideal. I was an audience member as well as a lecturer for their program. Some years later I would participate and perform surgery on neglected clubfeet on their mission trips to Honduras. This group currently continues its service to the underserved pediatric patients in Honduras and recently in India under the name Operation Footprint, Inc.

The persistent dogma throughout the involved community was that the clubfoot was a resistant congenital deformity that could not be readily corrected by manipulation and needed an early extensive surgical release.

THE CLUBFOOT REVOLUTION

Dr. Ignacio Ponseti, MD lived a fascinating, circuitous life from graduating medical school in Barcelona in 1936, to surviving the Spanish Civil War while providing fracture

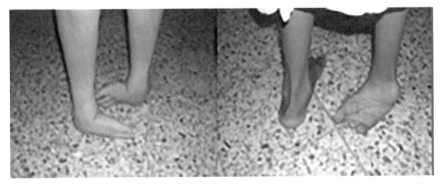

Fig. 9. A neglected clubfoot presenting in teenaged patients is commonly encountered on mission trips abroad.

and wound care to the injured. He then escaped to France while transporting wounded soldiers to safety. Seeking refuge, he then went to Mexico and began practicing rural medicine before finally going to Iowa City to train with Dr. Arthur Steindler in 1941 in the Orthopedic Department at the now named University of Iowa. He questioned the possibility of a better treatment method for clubfeet after seeing the results of extensive surgeries on these feet leaving them rigid, weak, painful, full of cicatrix, and poorly functioning.

He dissected clubfeet of stillborn babies to obtain an understanding of the true patho-anatomy of the rearfoot deformity. He developed a manipulation technique in 1948 that effectively corrected the deformity with serial casting and a percutaneous Achilles tenotomy. This was maintained by the use of brace consisting of shoes attached to a bar for a period of time to prevent relapses. He published an article in 1963 that demonstrated satisfactory results in a group of 67 patients utilizing this non-operative method.[18] In 1972, another excellent article was published showing his understanding of the clubfoot anatomy including the dissection pictures and the precise manipulation steps that produces these excellent results.[19] However, he continued to perform miracles on many patients in relative obscurity in Iowa, and his articles and results went largely unnoticed by the surgical community. However, many families seeking an alternative to the extensive and costly surgery with notably poor results were increasingly traveling to Iowa to be treated. Extensive posterior medial release continued to be performed exclusively for clubfoot worldwide.

DEVELOPING THE KAISER CONNECTION

In the late 1990's, Dr Ponseti made several trips to the San Francisco Bay Area to follow-up with many of his patients living here who had made the trek to Iowa City and were treated there previously. I and a colleague, Michael Colburn, DPM, were very privileged to have him visit our clinic in the Permanente Medical Group facility in Pleasanton and train us in his technique (**Fig. 10**). He was very excited with our understanding of the axis of the subtalar joint, the motions of the rearfoot, and our realization that holding the calcaneus during manipulation(Kite's mistake) actually blocked the reduction of the deformity. The whole concept clicked when I saw him put his

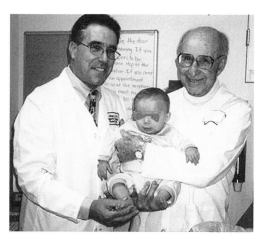

Fig. 10. Dr. Ponseti held an in-service teaching his technique at the Pleasanton clinic in the late 1990's.

thumb on the lateral head of the talus, push up on the first ray, supinate, and abduct the foot into correction (**Fig. 11**). The foot easily rotated out around the talus opening up the talo-calcaneal angle and everting the calcaneus. With a few casts, he corrected a foot on one of my patients who was then in plaster and had been scheduled for forthcoming surgery. I will never forget him softly singing lullabies in Spanish that instantly calmed even the most agitated, squirming infant. This was one part of his technique that I couldn't reproduce! This was a game-changing revelation to see the amazing effects of simply changing hand positions during manipulation. I was forever a believer in his technique and would strictly apply it to all my subsequent patients for the duration of my practice.

I soon understood that the calcaneus couldn't dorsiflex with the tenotomy until the foot was fully abducted and the calcaneus had moved out from underneath the talus. This is why the tenotomy is not performed until the foot is fully abducted past 60° externally, or at least until the anterosuperior process is felt out from underneath the talar head laterally, particularly in the complex clubfoot. Performing this too soon is doomed to failure. He patiently instructed us how to perform the tenotomy, although he didn't like our use of a #67 blade.

His West Coast patients held a reunion in the Kaiser in Pleasanton, CA and celebrated his birthday by presenting him with a special quilt containing the names of the many children he had cured. I was inspired by the seeing the long-term excellent results of these fully functioning patients and the admiration and appreciation on the parents' faces as they celebrated with their guru. Many children literally were dancing and showing off their feet as a tribute to this incredible pioneer. All of this correction with resulting normal function was without the routine extensive surgical release, which heretofore been considered standard.

In 2000, I accompanied Dr Ponseti to the Tachdjian's Pediatric Orthopedic International Seminar in San Francisco. At the conference, we proudly sat in the front row and a prominent speaker (remaining unnamed) leaned forward toward us and stated that clubfoot was purely a surgical deformity, and there was logically no way that a conservative treatment of manipulation and casting could ever fully work. After what miracles I had just previously seen during the in-services, I looked at Dr. Ponseti, and he gave me a knowing smile and shrugged off the criticism.

The belated and almost universal acceptance of the Ponseti technique was due to two main reasons. In the 1990's, he came out of retirement to treat more patients, educate more practitioners who would spend time in Iowa and published an easy to

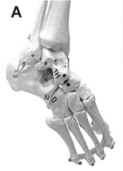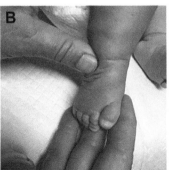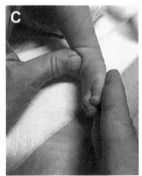

Fig. 11. (*A*) The thumb is placed on the lateral talar head, (*B*) the first ray is elevated and (*C*) and the foot supinated and abducted around the talus with the calcaneus everting from underneath the talus.

follow textbook summarizing the technique and results of his 50 yearlong life's passion[20] (**Fig. 12**). This increased interest in his method set the stage for its current worldwide universal acceptance. The literature soon became filled with many peer-reviewed studies and case reviews (too numerous to cite here) documenting and confirming his high rate of reproducible and excellent results, its safety, and cost effectiveness.

The second reason was the advent of the Internet which provided families seeking more conservative treatment for their infants with clubfeet a means of communicating and sharing their experience and knowledge of physicians who were proficient in the Ponseti technique. These forums united parents in the belief that major surgery should be avoided at all costs for clubfoot treatment, and they should seek conservative care. One of the first sites I saw was a Yahoo chat room titled "NoSurgery4Clubfoot" which began to turn the tide in favor of the Ponseti method. Parents demanded this method and they would leave your office and seek treatment elsewhere if not offered or they felt that you were not familiar with technique.

The rest is history and the Ponseti method became universally recognized as the preferred treatment of care and has been accepted globally. Its efficacy and outcomes are universal. The documentations are too extensive to list but are readily available for your perusal. One confirmatory case series came from our own institution in 2003[21] Internet sites and how to instructional videos proliferated. The gold standard is the Ponseti International Association (www.ponseti.info) based at the University of Iowa, which contains a wealth of information and instructions for both parents and practitioners alike.

REFINING A CLUBFOOT PRACTICE AT KAISER PERMANENTE

I submitted case documentations, pre and posttreatment clinical photographs, including my thumb position on the plaster casts and progression of abduction and

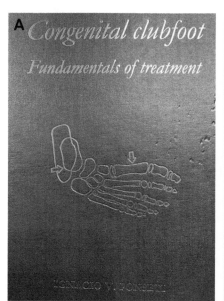 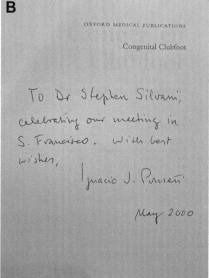

Fig. 12. The definitive textbook that changed the way that clubfoot is treated universally. (*A*) The cover and (*B*) the title page.

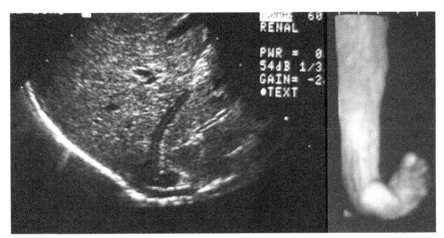

Fig. 13. This prenatal ultrasound demonstrating a clubfoot would prompt a genetics referral and a podiatric consultation for discussion of its treatment. However, a positional turned in foot wasn't always a true clubfoot needed manipulation.

final correction to the Ponseti International Association for their evaluation. After I became a recognized practitioner, I soon had patients from all over the northern California region seeking my expertise. Many were "doctor shopping" after becoming aware of a clubfoot seen on routine prenatal ultrasound (**Fig. 13**). They wanted assurance that surgery would not be performed and were willing to travel great distances to

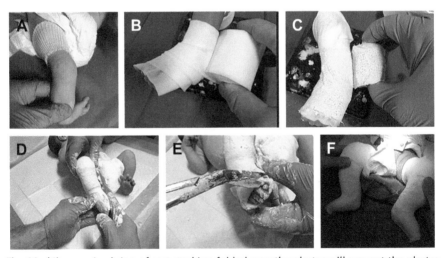

Fig. 14. (A) a proximal ring of cast stocking folded over the plaster will prevent the plaster irritation of the thigh. (B) apply very thin padding overlapping by one-half to allow accurate plaster molding. (C) soak extra fast set plaster 2 inch rolls in hot water and roll fast and low, do not lift the roll off of the leg or it will banana(unroll). (D) apply below knee (BK) portion first, mold thoroughly, and increase correction, including a pocket posteriorly to capture the heel, apply anterior knee slab then complete the above knee (AK) section. (E) trim dorsally to allow extensor function. (F) the foot is ready for the tenotomy when fully abducted past 60° external rotation.

receive the Ponseti method. We were very happy to accommodate them but soon recognized systems issues with scheduling.

It soon became apparent that working-in a time intense clubfoot infant to a normal busy clinic schedule was dysfunctional. These patients needed a specialized and compassionate cast removal by a gentle orthopedic technician, a weight check, washing, and lotion application of the legs, before manipulation into correction and a careful cast application (**Fig. 14**). Significantly more time was needed for the tenotomy procedure (**Fig. 15**). This was extremely time-consuming, stressful, and disruptive to a normal day. My chief was extremely accommodating, and a weekly, half

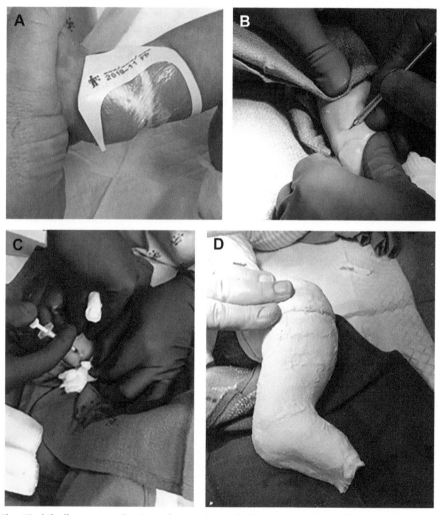

Fig. 15. (A) allow an application of topical anesthetic cream under occlusion to numb the skin for 20 to 30min.(while the procedure room is being set up). (B) palpate the Achilles tendon medial border, insert a #67 blade parallel and just anterior to the tendon, then rotate 90, feel a snap when completely severed. Be aware of the proximity of the peroneal artery (C). now inject the local anesthetic, could not feel the tendon contour if instilled pre-tenotomy. (D) the fully abducted and dorsiflexed cast is left on for 3 weeks.

day clinic was set up exclusively for the clubfoot patients. A resident was usually present to help and be educated in this technique. A dedicated orthopedic technician who loved babies helped with the casting and calmed the infant during tenotomies. We developed and kept handy an illustrated manual depicting the set-up for both casting and the tenotomies. Any medical assistant could easily and correctly prepare the room for these patients. A procedure room was normally used for the tenotomies, although many were performed on a standard exam chair/table. The infant was never taken to the OR for the tenotomy.

Initially, the protocol was to have the infant wear the shoes attached to abduction braces for a decreasing amount of hours per day until just 12 hours at age 1 year. This was continued until 2 years of age or so when the brace was discontinued. There were some relapses which were corrected with a percutaneous Achilles tenotomy and an anterior tibialis transfer under the retinaculum into the lateral cuneiform at a later age. These problems were significantly decreased when the brace was worn for 4 or more years at night. The newer, more comfortable shoes and articulated braces greatly increased parent compliance with their use. The main factor leading to relapse was the failure to use the night splint for the proper length of time.[22,23] I routinely emphasized to the parents starting with the first visit, "the only thing that you can do wrong is to not use the bar" (**Fig. 16**). Also, there are cute videos available online showing babies in bars, developing normally and reinforcing the need for consistent usage and that it doesn't interfere their activities.

A clubfoot is a whole limb deformity that may develop slightly shorter and appear thinner than a normal one. This was more apparent with the previous method of treatment with its prolonged cast immobilization, but still can be seen even with properly performed Ponseti technique..[24,25] It, therefore, is always very important initially to inform the parents of a potential size discrepancy, especially when the clubfoot is unilateral (**Fig. 17**).

There was another benefit to having all clubfoot patients scheduled on a specific day beside efficiency. This was the support group atmosphere of having many babies and their parents in the waiting room at the same time. They shared their experiences, progress, and outcomes congenially. They exchanged tips on shoe and brace wear and accessories while encouraging each other to be compliant. We routinely applied a topical anesthetic cream to the tenotomy site over the Achilles tendon and had the patient return to the waiting room to allow numbing for a period of time. Often, the other parents would clap when this infant re-emerged after the procedure in a show of support, gratitude, and relief.

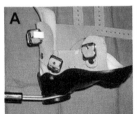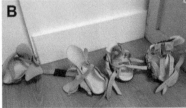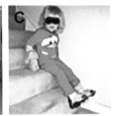

Fig. 16. Various types of user friendly shoes and braces are currently available. Parental non compliance with brace usage until 4 years of age has been directly correlated with poorer outcomes. (*A*) The clubfoot shoe is attached to the bar and set 60 degrees externally, (*B*) parental non compliance with proper bar usage until 4 years of age is correlated with poorer outcomes and (*C*) older children must refrain from ambulating when wearing the bar.

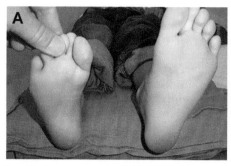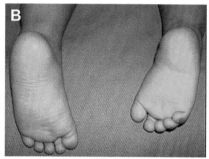

Fig. 17. Parents must be initially made aware that limb length discrepancies, leg girth differences and smaller feet are common in unilateral deformities, despite proper treatment as seen in these (*A*) plantar and (*B*) dorsal views.

SUMMARY

This article chronicles my clubfoot treatment transition over the decades from extensive posterior medial soft tissue release surgery to the total adoption of the Ponseti method. The current results are overwhelmingly excellent producing lasting functional feet without significant disability in the long term. This technique works best when performed exactly as described by Dr Ponseti and strict adherence to the protocol.[26,27]

CLINICS CARE POINTS

- The Kite method of manipulation was historically used to treat clubfeet. After a period of casting, an extensive posterior medial surgical soft tissue release was performed to realign the foot. The results were less than satisfactory and often multiple further surgeries were necessary as the child developed.

- Dr Ponseti pioneered a method of manipulation, casting, and percutaneous Achilles tenotomy that effectively corrected these feet without the need for extensive surgery.

- The Ponseti method has been universally accepted globally and is the standard of care for the treatment of clubfeet.

DISCLOSURE

None.

REFERENCES

1. Kite JH. The clubfoot. New York: Grune and Stratton; 1964.
2. Turco VJ. Resistant congenital club foot–one-stage posteromedial release with internal fixation. A follow-up report of a fifteen-year experience. J Bone Joint Surg Am 1979;61(6A):805–14.
3. Karlin JM. The Cincinnati incision. A new surgical approach for clubfoot and ankle surgery. J Am Podiatr Med Assoc 1986;76(7):386–9. https://doi.org/10.7547/87507315-76-7-386.
4. Lehman WB. The clubfoot. Philadelphia: J. B. Lippincott; 1980.
5. Turco VJ. Clubfoot. New York: Churchill Livingston; 1981.
6. Devalentine SJ. Foot and ankle Disorders in children. New York: Churchill Livingston; 1992.

7. Simons GW. The clubfoot: the present and a View of the future. New York: Springer-Verlag; 1994.
8. Green AD, Lloyd-Roberts GC. The results of early posterior release in resistant club feet. A long-term review. J Bone Joint Surg Br 1985;67(4):588–93.
9. Hutchins PM, Foster BK, Paterson DC, et al. Long-term results of early surgical release in club feet. J Bone Joint Surg Br 1985;67(5):791–9.
10. Ippolito E, Farsetti P, Caterini R, et al. Long-term comparative results in patients with congenital clubfoot treated with two different protocols. J Bone Joint Surg Am 2003;85(7):1286–94.
11. Cummings RJ, Bashore CJ, Bookout CB, et al. Avascular necrosis of the talus after McKay clubfoot release for idiopathic congenital clubfoot. J Pediatr Orthop 2001;21(2):221–4.
12. Hootnick DR, Packard DS Jr, Levinsohn EM, et al. Ischemic necrosis following clubfoot surgery: the purple hallux sign. J Pediatr Orthop B 2004;13(5):315–22.
13. Hootnick DR, Packard DS Jr, Levinsohn EM. Necrosis leading to amputation following clubfoot surgery. Foot Ankle 1990;10(6):312–6.
14. Weseley MS, Barenfeld PA, Barrett N. Complications of the treatment of clubfoot. Clin Orthop Relat Res 1972;84:93–6.
15. McKay DW. New concept of and approach to clubfoot treatment: section II–correction of the clubfoot. J Pediatr Orthop 1983;3(1):10–21.
16. Noonan KJ, Meyers AM, Kayes K. Leg length discrepancy in unilateral congenital clubfoot following surgical treatment. Iowa Orthop J 2004;24:60–4.
17. Blakeslee TJ, DeValentine SJ. Management of the resistant idiopathic clubfoot: the Kaiser experience from 1980-1990. J Foot Ankle Surg 1995;34(2):167–76.
18. Ponseti IV, Smoley EN. The classic: congenital club foot: the results of treatment. 1963. Clin Orthop Relat Res 2009;467(5):1133–45.
19. Ponseti IV, Campos J. The classic: observations on pathogenesis and treatment of congenital clubfoot. 1972. Clin Orthop Relat Res 2009;467(5):1124–32.
20. Ponseti IV. Congenital clubfoot. Fundamentals of treatment. New York: Oxford University Press; 1996.
21. Colburn M, Williams M. Evaluation of the treatment of idiopathic clubfoot by using the Ponseti method. J Foot Ankle Surg 2003;42(5):259–67.
22. Ponseti IV. Common errors in the treatment of congenital clubfoot. Int Orthop 1997;21(2):137–41.
23. Dobbs MB, Rudzki JR, Purcell DB, et al. Factors predictive of outcome after use of the Ponseti method for the treatment of idiopathic clubfeet. J Bone Joint Surg Am 2004;86(1):22–7.
24. Fulton Z, Briggs D, Silva S, et al. Calf circumference discrepancies in patients with unilateral clubfoot: Ponseti versus surgical release. J Pediatr Orthop 2015; 35(4):403–6.
25. Shimode K, Miyagi N, Majima T, et al. Limb length and girth discrepancy of unilateral congenital clubfeet. J Pediatr Orthop B 2005;14(4):280–4.
26. Miller NH, Carry PM, Mark BJ, et al. Does strict adherence to the Ponseti method Improve isolated clubfoot treatment outcomes? A two-institution review. Clin Orthop Relat Res 2016;474(1):237–43.
27. Zhao D, Li H, Zhao L, et al. Results of clubfoot management using the Ponseti method: do the details matter? A systematic review. Clin Orthop Relat Res 2014;472(4):1329–36.
28. Ponseti IV, Zhivkov M, Davis N, et al. Treatment of the complex idiopathic clubfoot. Clin Orthop Relat Res 2006;451:171–6.

Clubfoot

Emphasis on the Complex and Atypical Subsets

Mitzi L. Williams, DPM, FACFAS, FACFAP[a],*,
Matthew B. Dobbs, MD, FACS, FAAOS, FAOA[b,c,d,e,f]

KEYWORDS

- Clubfoot • Atypical clubfoot • Complex clubfoot • Ponseti • Clubfoot casting
- Talipes equinovarus • Congenital foot deformity • Pediatric orthopedics

KEY POINTS

- Congenital clubfoot (talipes equinovarus) is a complex multiplanar deformity involving cavus, adductus, varus, and equinus.
- The Ponseti method has proven to be successful in the treatment of both isolated and nonisolated clubfoot.
- Atypical clubfoot, which is mistakenly used synonymously with complex clubfoot, is a different entity though the casting treatment and technique is the same as it is for complex clubfoot.
- The atypical subset is associated with neurologic and or motor deficits.

DEFINITION

Congenital clubfoot (talipes equinovarus) is a complex multiplanar deformity involving cavus, adductus, varus, and equinus. While a variety of deformities can present in infancy clubfoot is truly defined by its hindfoot varus deformity in association with equinus. The condition affects 1 out of every 1000 live births with a male-to-female ratio of 2:1.[1] It remains one of the most common birth defects, which can be isolated or of neurologic influence. While many are isolated birth defects, approximately 20% are linked to neuromuscular and/or genetic conditions. Specifically, mutations in the PITX1-TBX4-HOXC transcriptional pathway have been noted to cause familial clubfoot and vertical talus in a small number of families.[2] In children, 50% present bilaterally.

[a] Kaiser San Francisco Bay Area Foot and Ankle Residency Program, Department of Orthopedics and Podiatric Surgery, Kaiser Permanente, 3600 Broadway, Oakland, CA 94611, USA; [b] Palm Beach International Surgery Center, Paley Institute, 5325 Greenwood Avenue, Suite 203, West Palm Beach, FL 33407, USA; [c] Clinical Orthopaedics and Related Research; [d] United States Bone and Joint Initiative; [e] Association of Bone and Joint Surgeons; [f] International Federation of Pediatric Orthopaedic Societies
* Corresponding author. 3600 Broadway Suite 17, Oakland, CA 94611.
E-mail address: Mitzi.L.Williams@kp.org

Clin Podiatr Med Surg 41 (2024) 17–25
https://doi.org/10.1016/j.cpm.2023.06.009
0891-8422/24/© 2023 Elsevier Inc. All rights reserved.

Hawaiians and Maoris have been reported to have the greatest prevalence at 7 per 1000 live births.[1,3] (**Fig. 1**)

HISTORY

Clubfoot treatment has undergone transformation over the last three decades. Kite was the first in the United States to have his non-operative treatment protocol accepted, with a series of manipulation and casting.[4] However, many cases of club-feet were still treated operatively. While Kite encouraged a noninvasive manipulation, his method was faulty. Counterpressure on the calcaneocuboid joint blocked the migration of the calcaneus from being able to move from a varus position to a more valgus position beneath the talus. Over the last few decades, there has been a para-digmatic shift in the treatment of clubfoot, due to the work of Dr. Ignacio Ponseti.[5,6]

As the son of a watchmaker, Dr. Ignacio Ponseti, was accustomed to working with delicate small components. He was further given the opportunity as a physician to perform retrospective reviews of children who had undergone posteromedial releases and surgical reconstructions at an early age. He concluded these young children had developed stiff, under corrected, and often painful feet. Likewise, their function was compromised.[7–9] Not only did he study these children from a functional standpoint, but he also studied them on a cellular level.

From a histopathologic standpoint, he concluded that many children with clubfoot, when operated on especially under the age of one, had developed an abundance of scar tissue, an increase in collagen fibrils, and retracting fibrosis, which led to recurrence of the deformity.[10] These microscopic and macroscopic findings led him to the development of a less invasive approach. He developed the Ponseti approach for management of clubfoot and confirmed its success by long-term follow up studies.[5,11]

The Ponseti method is now the first line of treatment for the management of both idiopathic/isolated clubfoot while it is also the accepted first line of treatment for the

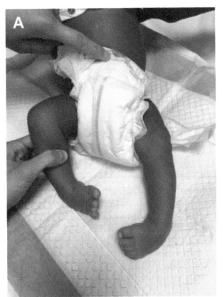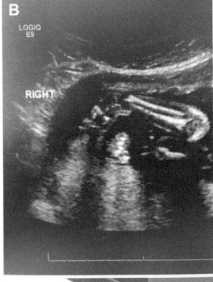

Fig. 1. (*A*) Clubfoot deformity demonstrating cavus, adductus, varus and equinus (*B*) Suspected clubfoot on ultrasound in utero.

syndromic/nonisolated clubfoot.[12] Numerous studies demonstrate the effectiveness of the Ponseti method and need for subsequent bracing compliance until the minimum age of 4 years.[5,11] Poor bracing utilization is the greatest reason for recurrence.[13] Following the Ponseti method, boots and an abduction bar brace must be utilized as recurrent equinus, inversion, and or adduction can occur. Upon recurrence, the Ponseti method is still valuable in reducing deformity while 40% of the clubfoot population will require some form of surgery for the management of clubfoot in their lifetime.[2,14] (**Fig. 2**).

ANATOMY OF CLUBFOOT

Untreated clubfoot has profound effects on gait and function. The goal of treatment is to obtain a stable, plantigrade foot with mobility. If untreated, the deformity becomes much more difficult to treat conservatively, and worsens over time. Patients may have little or even no pain during ambulation, but will undoubtedly develop abnormal, thickened skin and bursae on the dorsolateral foot. Children with untreated clubfeet are often unable to wear shoe gear. Weakness of the lower extremity and a smaller calf size may decrease the ability to participate in high impact activity. Since the talus and calcaneus are notably plantarflexed, there is an equinus gait and compensation that occurs with knee hyperextension and hip external rotation. There is also an increase in knee and hip joint moments and decrease in ankle moments, likely due to weak calf muscles and plantarflexors. A weak posterior muscle group can lead to decreased push-off strength. Complete foot drop may also occur due to the overall foot architecture.

Conservative treatment using the Ponseti technique has provided a functional, plantigrade foot in 85% to 95% of patients.[6,10,11,15–17] It has been reported that even after treatment there is decreased ankle range of motion when compared to unaffected

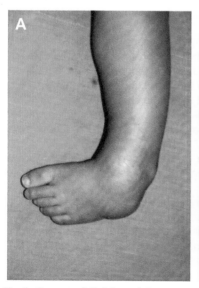 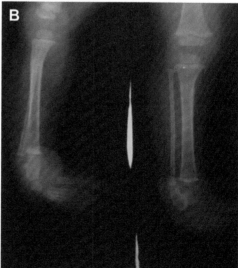

Fig. 2. Untreated Clubfoot: (*A*) One notes the enlarged bursa lateral foot in which is loaded during ambulation. The head of the talus is laterally deviated and in malalignment within the ankle mortise. The hindfoot remains in varus and equinus. The calcaneus never migrated beneath the talus out of varus. (*B*) X-rays of untreated clubfoot.

children, but overall, there is increased ankle range of motion and strength, as well as less pain after casting.[18] This is accompanied by decreased peak pressures over the medial forefoot and hindfoot as well as increased pressure over the lateral midfoot. Residual intoeing is seen in up to 33% of children with moderate clubfoot using the Dimeglio scoring system.[19] Normal ankle sagittal plane motion may be obtained using casting or physical therapy in children with severe clubfoot, and almost two-thirds of patients have normal kinematic ankle motion if treated properly.[19,20] The previous article of this book is dedicated to the history and current treatment of idiopathic/isolated clubfoot. Here we further the discussion of the complex and atypical clubfoot subsets.

TREATMENT

The Ponseti method has proven to be successful in the treatment of both isolated and nonisolated clubfoot. The method should be executed prior to any pediatric invasive procedures and likewise should be attempted with any pediatric recurrence.[14] Quite often, the method provides a stretch and can improve overall foot position minimizing procedures needed to obtain a plantigrade foot. Still, it is important to recognize that without proper bracing following serial casting recurrence is likely at a time of growth.[13] Despite the methods, effectiveness 40% of children will require some form of surgical intervention in their lifetime.[2,14] Proper use of the method can minimize the extent of procedures required or eliminate the need for surgery. The use of the Ponseti method for the treatment of relapses has too proven to be helpful in minimizing surgical procedures needed.

The Ponseti Method
- A full musculoskeletal examination is performed prior to treatment.
- The Magic Move: A dorsiflexory force is applied beneath the 1st metatarsal head with counterpressure applied to the lateral talar head. This maneuver reduces the cavus and medial crease. This is performed, as the forefoot is not as inverted as compared to the hindfoot.
- Do not touch the calcaneus or cuboid during manipulations.
- Upon the resolution of the medial crease, the forefoot is abducted with counterpressure applied to the lateral talar head. Upon the reduction of the adduction, inversion, and cavus one can proceed with the correction of the equinus.
- A complete Achilles tenotomy is performed to reduce equinus if less than 10° of dorsiflexion is noted at the level of the ankle joint. A final cast is applied and left intact for 2 to 3 weeks. The vast majority of children do need this tenotomy to be performed.
- Abduction bar bracing is utilized until age 4 at minimum. The affected foot is externally rotated at 50 to 70° to the lower leg and an unaffected foot is positioned to 30 to 40° to the lower limb.
- The need for patient-focused bracing strategies is a topic for research.
- The use of an abduction dorsiflexion mechanism (ADM) as compared to the boot/abduction bar bracing can be helpful in the older child with recurrences or the young child with proximal knee and hip contractures.
- It is important to evaluate children individually (**Fig. 3**).

Casting Pearls
- A thin layer of webril or cast padding is utilized from the toes up to the groin.
- A well-molded plaster cast is utilized and secured from the toes to just below the knee. Once completed, plaster is continued above the knee while maintaining 90 to 110° of knee flexion to minimize cast slippage.

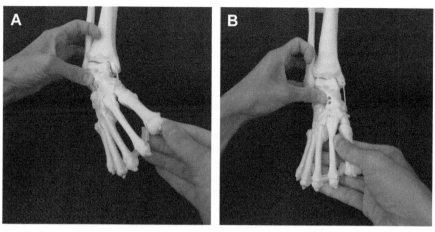

Fig. 3. The Ponseti method: (*A*) Dorsiflexory force beneath the first metatarsal head, (*B*) Abduction of the forefoot with counterpressure on the lateral talar head.

- Excess plaster is removed to expose the toes.
- Semi rigid casting material may be utilized in place of plaster while proper manipulation and molding is key (**Fig. 4**).

Casting Pitfalls

- Improper manipulation and or forceful manipulation in casts
- Inappropriate pressure applied to calcaneus

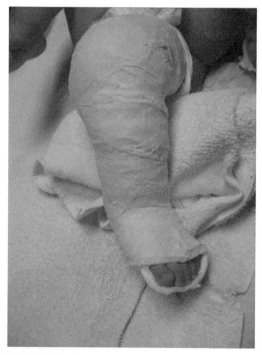

Fig. 4. Ponseti casting for clubfoot.

- Counterpressure to the calcaneocuboid joint
- Excessive cast padding
- Removal of casts prior to appointment
- Failure to recognize complex or atypical clubfoot subsets

Complex clubfoot

Complex clubfoot is used to describe a type of clubfoot that is more resistant to standard casting technique and develops a distinct phenotype during the casting process. This type of clubfoot is usually not recognized at birth as being different. Often, correction ceases to occur in the middle of the casting series and the foot becomes short, fat, with a retracted first ray. Cast slipping is common, and, if it occurs, a deep plantar crease is evident indicating worsening cavus. Fortunately, Ponseti recognized this entity and developed modified casting technique to correct that is extremely effective. The emphasis is on dorsiflexing the first and 5th ray to stretch the plantar crease. Serial casts result in achieving 30 to 40° of external rotation. At that time a tenotomy is done and the foot is casted in 50° of external rotation and 10° of dorsiflexion. Trying to externally rotate the foot further results in a midfoot breach laterally. Hyperflexion of the knee up to 110° is helpful to prevent slipping. Care should be taken to use a posterior plaster slab for the lower leg and dorsal slab for the knee to minimize the amount of plaster rolls. This too assists with deformity correction. This technique leads to better molding. Foot abduction bracing is used after the casting, but care should be taken to set the feet at 50° of external rotation and not greater. Children, if corrected, can perform very well functionally with lower risks of recurrence as compared to the atypical clubfoot subset. The complex clubfoot is one which can develop secondary to cast slippage and faulty maneuvers.

The Complex Clubfoot (21)
- May present with deep plantar crease initially and extreme cavus. Hyperabduction may lead to the tightening of the quadratus plantae and pulling of the flexors. This leads to worsening cavus.
- Resistant to classic Ponseti Method
- Often identified around the time of the second cast
- This condition can be the result of improper manipulation and casting. Cast slippage can be associated with the complex subset.
- The 4-finger technique is utilized: Pushing upwards beneath the 1st and 5th metatarsals while applying a dorsiflexory force on the posterior superior aspect of the calcaneus (**Fig. 5**).

Atypical clubfoot

Atypical clubfoot, which is mistakenly used synonymously with complex clubfoot, is a different entity though the casting treatment and technique is the same as it is for complex clubfoot. (21) Atypical clubfeet share many of the same clinical features as complex clubfoot, but these are identifiable at birth with a good physical examination. Patients with atypical clubfeet have weak or absent active dorsiflexion of the toes and ankle as well as weak active eversion of the foot. This subset is associated with neurologic and or motor deficits. The physician must be mindful that a formal neurologic diagnosis may not be present in infancy. While arthrogryposis and myelomeningocele are commonly associated with the atypical subset children may have isolated weakness of various compartments without a diagnosed syndrome. Casting is done as for complex clubfoot, but these patients are at higher risk of relapse due to lack of motor strength and often neurologic influence.

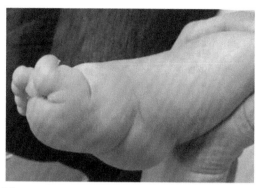

Fig. 5. Complex clubfoot.

Atypical Clubfoot
- Noted at birth
- Weak or absent active dorsiflexion of the toes and ankle as well as weak active eversion of the foot
- Associated with neurologic and/or motor deficits
- Deep plantar crease initially and extreme cavus. Hyperabduction may lead to the tightening of the quadratus plantae and pulling of the flexors. This leads to worsening cavus.
- Resistant to classic Ponseti method
- The 4-finger technique is utilized: Pushing upwards beneath the 1st and 5th metatarsals while applying a dorsiflexory force on the posterior superior aspect of the calcaneus
- Higher risks of relapse given motor strength deficit

BRACING PERIOD

In many ways the bracing period can be much more challenging for parents and families as compared to casting. There is always a feeling of accomplishment and relief amongst parents upon the completion of casts. The break in period for braces can come as a surprise. It is important to educate all caregivers on the importance of bracing and the high risks for the recurrence of clubfoot without proper bracing utilization. Immediately following the casting period, the child transitions to boots attached to an abduction bar. It is important to educate caregivers that while the braces do not cause pain they are a change, especially for an infant.

Children who have proximal joint contractures may benefit from other bracing modalities such as the abduction dorsiflexion mechanism brace (ADM) to minimize any worsening proximal joint deformities. This brace serves a role in assisting older children who are status post serial casting and or surgical procedures for the management of recurrences.

SUMMARY

Clubfoot continues to be one of the most common congenital musculoskeletal conditions treated worldwide. Through research, the Ponseti technique has proven over the years to be the first-line treatment in congenital clubfoot. It remains essential to be accurate with this approach while too performing a thorough neurologic examination throughout the care of each child. This will continue to help in the identification of the atypical subset and need for this specific maneuver to obtain deformity correction. Despite care some children will need more in their lifetime. Long-term follow-up while the child grows will help minimize progressive rigid deformities. Individualized care should be the focus.

CLINICS CARE POINTS

- With every examination one should evaluate for weakness or motor deficits. Often in infancy a formal neurologic diagnosis or syndrome may not be established.
- This weakness should raise the suspicion of an atypical clubfoot subset and need for this specific approach. The clinical appearance of the foot is key.
- A transverse crease separating the heel from the remainder of the foot is quite different than the more classic medial crease.
- Weakness of the toes should be noted. One should highlight these findings and to have a higher suspicion for an atypical subset. While deformity correction is key, one should not cause a subsequent deformity.

DISCLOSURE

A co author is an inventor of the Dobbs Bars.

REFERENCES

1. Chung CS, Nemechek RW, Larsen IJ, et al. Genetic and epidemiological studies of clubfoot in Hawaii. General and medical considerations. Hum Hered 1969;19: 321–42.
2. Dobbs MB, Gurnett CA. The 2017 ABJS nicolas Andry Award: Advancing personalized medicine for clubfoot through translational research. Clin Orthop Relat Res 2017;475:1716–25.
3. Beals RK. Club foot in the Maori: a genetic study of 50 kindres. N Z Med J 1978; 88:144–6.
4. Kite JH. The clubfoot. New York: Grune & Sttatton; 1964.
5. Cooper DM, Dietz FR. Treatment of idiopathic clubfoot. A thirty- year follow- up note. J Bone Joint Surg Am 1995;77:1477–89.
6. Ponseti IV. Treatment of congenital clubfoot. J Bone Joint Surg Am 1992;74(3): 448–54.
7. Ippolito E. Update on pathological anatomy of clubfoot. J Pediatr Orthop 1995;4: 17–24.
8. Ippolito E, Ponseti IV. Congential clubfoot in the human fetus. A histological study. J Bone Joint Surg Am 1980;62:8–22.
9. Dobbs MB, Nunley R, Schoenecker PL. Long-term follow up of patients with clubfoot treated with extensive soft tissue release. J Bone Joint Surg Am 2006;88:986–96.
10. Ponseti IV. Congenital clubfoot: fundamentals of treatment. Oxford University Press; 1996.
11. Laaveg SJ, Ponseti IV. Long-term results of treatment of congenital clubfoot. J Bone Joint Surg Am 1980;62(1):23–31.
12. Arkin C, Ihnow S, Dias L, et al. Midterm results of the Ponseti method for treatment of clubfoot in patients with spina bifida. J Pediatr Orthop 2018;38(10): e588–92.

13. Dobbs MB, Rudzki JR, Purcell DB, et al. Factors predictive of outcome after use of the Ponseti methods for the treatment of idiopathic clubfoot. J Bone Joint Surg 2004;86-A(No1).
14. van Praag VM, Lysenko M, Harvey B, et al. Casting is effective for recurrence following Ponseti treatment of clubfoot. J Bone Joint Surg Am 2018;100:1001–8.
15. Abdelgawad AA, Lehman WB, van Bosse HJ, et al. Treatment of idiopathic clubfoot using the Ponseti method: minimum 2-year follow-up. J Pediatr Orthop B 2007;16(2):98–105.
16. Bor N, Coplan JA, Herzenberg JE. Ponseti treatment for idiopathic clubfoot: minimum 5-year followup. Clin Orthop Relat Res 2008;467(5):1263–70.
17. Banskota B, Yadav P, Rajbhandari T, et al. Outcomes of the Ponseti method for untreated clubfeet in Nepalese patients seen between the ages of one and five years and followed for at least 10 years. J Bone Joint Surg Am 2018;100:2004–14.
18. Sinclair MF, Bosch K, Rosenbaum D, et al. Pedobarographic analysis following Ponseti treatment for congenital clubfoot. Clin Orthop Relat Res 2009;467: 1223–30.
19. Gottschalk HP, Karol LA, Jeans KA. Gait analysis of children treated for moderate clubfoot with physical therapy versus the Ponseti cast technique. J Pediatr Orthop 2010;30:235–9.
20. El-Hawary R, Karol LA, Jeans KA, et al. Gait analysis of children treated for clubfoot with physical therapy or the Ponseti cast technique. J Bone Joint Surg Am 2008;90:1508–16.

The Application of Morton's Observations to Contemporary Treatment of Foot Dysfunction

Lawrence Ford, DPM

KEYWORDS

- Evolution • Biomechanics • First ray • Medial column • Instability • Hypermobility
- Equinus • Propulsion

KEY POINTS

- Morton claimed that certain atavistic features are responsible for the etiology of the majority of foot complaints.
- Gastrocnemius equinus and first-ray hypermobility are remnants of an earlier stage in the evolution of the human foot and must be considered as causative factors in the development of postural foot pain.
- Foot balance depends on both the architectural structure of the bones and ligaments as well as postural strength afforded by the muscles. A deficit of either leads to an unbalanced foot.
- Lengthening of the gastrocsoleus complex and stabilization with realignment of the first ray should be considered critical components of the overall reconstruction of the foot.

INTRODUCTION

In 1935, Yale University anatomist Dudley J Morton published his seminal work identifying and analyzing the primary factors causing foot dysfunction. He produced a collection of studies and observations rooted in the understanding of human evolution and comparative primate anatomy.[1–3] The anatomy of the foot was proffered as strong evidence that humans originated from an arboreal environment. The musculoskeletal structure of the foot is strikingly similar to the hand and similar to the feet of our primate cousins and ancestors. It allowed for climbing and grasping, and subsequently evolved to facilitate weight-bearing locomotion on the ground. According to Morton, these atavistic features are responsible for the causes of the majority of foot complaints.[1–4] The term "Morton's foot" has been used to characterize this type of foot with traits related to an earlier stage in our evolution. In order to effectively treat

Kaiser San Francisco Bay Area Foot and Ankle Surgery, Department of Orthopedics and Podiatric Surgery, Kaiser Permanente, 3600 Broadway, Oakland, CA 94611, USA
E-mail address: lawrence.ford@kp.org

Clin Podiatr Med Surg 41 (2024) 27–41
https://doi.org/10.1016/j.cpm.2023.06.010
0891-8422/24/© 2023 Elsevier Inc. All rights reserved.

patients who exhibit these structural defects, it is important to understand their cause and effects on the human foot.

> The peculiar structure of the human foot, the arrangement and action of its muscles, its embryological changes, and the facts of comparative anatomy, can be explained in only one way-by presuming that there was a phase in man's history when he used his foot as a grasping climbing organ, much in the manner still retained by the arboreal chimpanzee.
>
> —Sir Arthur Keith, 1923.[5]

EARLY MAMMALIAN POSTURE

Early mammals developed a true heel that was ideal for climbing, in order to generate upward leverage against gravity. Muscle function around the heel and toes was differentiated. Digital muscles provided the ability to cling and grasp, whereas calcaneal muscles enabled upward leverage against body weight and gravity. Early tree dwelling mammals were quadrupedal. The midline axis of the foot was centered through the third metatarsal, which was the longest part of the forefoot and the fulcrum for leverage. Through brachiation, the upper extremities differentiated to become more adapt at swinging. The body took on a more vertical posture setting the stage for early bipedalism. The bones and muscles adapted with the progression of bipedal weight-bearing. This alteration affected every part of the skeletal structure, especially the foot. A lever requires structural rigidity, yet the foot of the early bipedal tree-dwelling mammal, which developed a vertical posture, was an ineffective and inefficient lever as it retained flexibility to grasp and support itself on branches. The forefoot differentiated itself into 2 grasping parts, the hallux on one side and the lateral metatarsals and digits on the other. This axis between the first and second rays provided an opposable hallux and lateral digits as well as support for an erect body structure. This change in the foot's axis from the third metatarsal in quadrupeds to between the first and second in bipeds is considered major evidence of the link between man and ape. It exists nowhere else in nature except as isolated, inconsistent anomalies.[1–4]

TERRESTRIAL ADAPTATIONS

In body structure, the gibbon represents the midway point between the more primitive, proanthropoid tree-living monkeys and the more advanced terrestrial, anthropoid apes. It is the most primitive of apes. It walks upright on the ground and on branches. Of the higher primates, the structure of the gorilla is the most similar to man (**Fig. 1**). Its foot has distinctly recognizable changes to its structure that are consistent with upright weight-bearing on the ground. These adaptations emerged as focus shifted from the upper extremities to the lower extremities, in particular the feet. Anatomical changes emerged, designed to aid in locomotion. Instead of prioritizing grasping, the digital muscles were used for structural stability, propulsion, and forward gait. The tarsal bones became more interlocked and therefore more efficient in producing work. This included the mortise articulation between the talus and lower leg, the talus becoming deeper and more of a press fit. One major change was depression of the heel to meet the ground. In order to stand upright with a balanced, erect posture, even distribution of weight between the front and back of the foot was required. The calcaneus had to bear weight to offer counter support for the metatarsals and digits. The posterior leg muscles had to elongate to allow this. Additionally, with conversion of the foot from a grasper to a lever used against body weight and gravity, the calcaneus became longer and larger. The tarsal bones of the gorilla add up to one-half

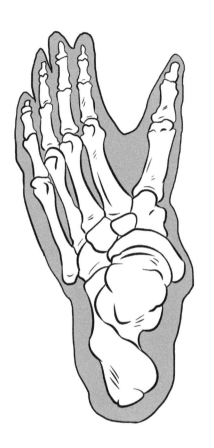 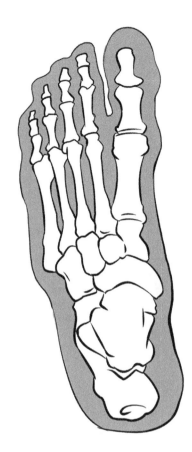

GORILLA   HUMAN

Fig. 1. Of the higher primates, the structure of the gorilla foot is most similar to man, reflecting the terrestrial modifications of upright posture and forward locomotion. The most notable difference is the along the medial column and first ray.

the length of the foot in contrast to the more arboreal chimpanzee, which only add up to one-third. The foot of the gorilla has notable changes that are characteristic of the human foot. Shorter lateral digits that are more plantarly directed toward the ground through torsional changes of the metatarsals reflect the terrestrial modifications adapted for support and upright forward motion. The early calcaneus had a plantar medially slanted sustentaculum tali similar to today's higher primates. Along with the navicular, it provided a ball and socket support for the talar head, although because of its obliquity, body weight and the longitudinal axis of the foot were deflected inwardly. The skewed concentration of load along the medial border of the foot created a flattening in the direction of pronation. With the calf muscle's action on the calcaneus to create a forward thrust on the foot, coupled with the slanted sustentaculum tali, the center of body weight was concentrated medially between the first and second metatarsals. The forefoot adapted a thicker, stouter first and second metatarsal in response, yet maintained a divergence in order to provide support, balance, and stability. In order for efficient gait though, the leverage axis (between the first and second metatarsals) needs to be parallel to the direction of travel. To accomplish this, the first metatarsal took on an even more important role as the subject of greater stress load, and adapted by enlarging and lengthening, altering the axis. By externally rotating the leg and closing the divergence between the first and second rays, the metatarsals were directed forward making the axis and direction of travel parallel. These changes are specific to the adoption of ground living habits. The foot as a stable lever trumped its importance as a grasper.[1–4]

DEVELOPMENT OF THE MEDIAL LONGITUDINAL ARCH

Wolff's law states that bones placed under stress will resist that stress by adapting and remodeling. The tensile stresses on the overloaded medial column of the foot would have been resisted by reactive compression stresses directed on the upper surface of the medial column. Morton proposed that this reactive remodeling lifted the depressed slant of the sustentaculum tali, which in turn lifted the talus in the direction of the leverage axis (**Fig. 2**). The net result of this was a redistribution of body weight to the lateral portion of the foot. Divergence of the hallux thus became a hindrance to more efficient forward leverage. With more lateral weight distribution and eventual convergence of the first ray, the first metatarsal needed to plantarflex at the midfoot enabling it to better resist the medial deflection of body weight.[1] This adaptation is reflected in the modern human foot as a parallel talar-first metatarsal axis (**Fig. 3**).

A   GORILLA   B   HUMAN

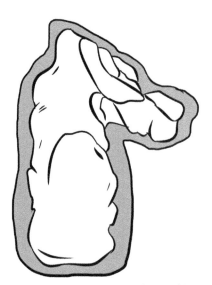
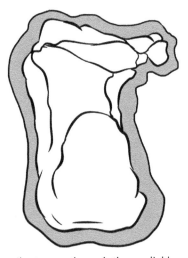

Fig. 2. The sustentaculum tali raised in response to tensile stresses through the medial longitudinal arch, transforming from an obliquely directed structure (*A*) to one that could resist depression of the talar head (*B*).

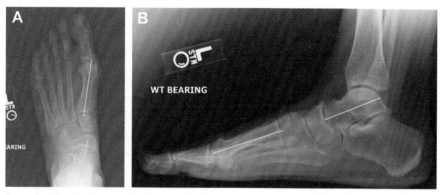

Fig. 3. (*A, B*) Adaptive changes to the foot because of weight-bearing with erect posture led to a stable first ray with a raised medial longitudinal arch. This is reflected in the modern human foot as a parallel talar–first metatarsal axis.

CENTER OF GRAVITY

In humans with erect posture, the center of gravity lies just anterior to the sacrum and the articulation of the hip. The increased size of the lower extremity skeleton, as a consequence of its increased importance, lowered the center of gravity to the level of the pelvis from its more proximal location in the gorilla and more anterior position in the Neanderthal man. With the center of gravity aligned with the body axis just anterior to the hip joint in erect posture, the legs became straight at the knee. This adjustment from a crouched posture like the gorilla to the fully erect posture of modern man required adaptation of the muscles of the leg such that minimal effort was required to stand erect (**Fig. 4**). Distally, body weight is centered through the talus at the tibiotalar joint. Center of gravity travels anterior to the ankle closer to the level of the navicular. This places increased work on the gastrocsoleus complex to stabilize and support this upright posture. This strain is easily compensated for by its size and mechanical advantage on the heel. As body weight is transmitted through the tibiotalar joint, the force placed on the arch of the foot is counteracted by the opposing pull of the calf muscle and by the plantar ligaments, including the plantar fascia, which transfers the stress to compression and subsequent stability of the medial longitudinal arch. By this mechanism, the foot evenly distributes body weight between the calcaneus and the metatarsals. The plantar ligaments of the foot have also adapted to their increased importance by becoming thicker and stronger. The ligaments retain some degree of flexibility in order to offer shock absorption, yet still provide resistance to the motion of the joints they buttress. Each metatarsal shares the load equally, although the first metatarsal carries twice the amount of each lesser metatarsal. The two sesamoids under the first metatarsal act as bearing points essentially dividing the load of the first metatarsal. The high point transversely is the base of the second metatarsal around which the medial and lateral forefoot is centered.[1,4]

LOCOMOTION AND GAIT

With forward locomotion, the center of gravity displaces anteriorly away from the center of body weight. The muscles that were in equilibrium in stance are converted into leverage action in order to propel the foot forward. In stance, the angle of gait is more lateral than in

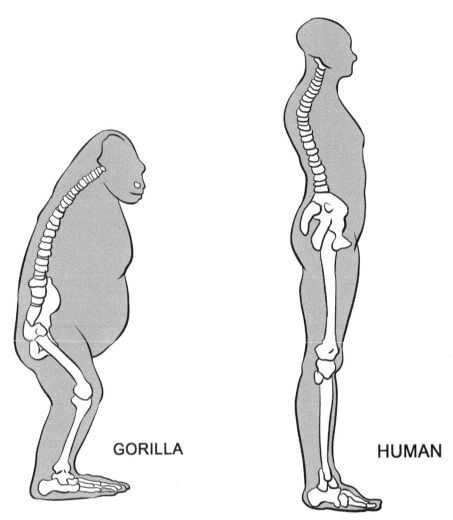

GORILLA   **HUMAN**

Fig. 4. Progression to a fully erect posture required lengthening of the posterior leg muscles. Morton suggested that tight calf muscles are an atavistic trait that causes uneven weight distribution across the foot.

walking, which is more lateral than in running. The angle of gait changes and is directly influenced by the hip in order to accommodate for postural stability versus forward locomotion. Abducting the foot and externally rotating the hip imparts stability and less muscular demand in stance. With faster walking and running, coordinated muscle demand is lessened with a narrower angle of gait. A mild degree of out-toeing is predominant, considered normal, and more efficient for gait. In weak or unbalanced feet, increased abduction can cause excessive strain on the medial border of the foot.[1,4]

There are two components of the weight-bearing phase of gait. One is gravitational. The foot reacts to the force of gravity on it. The other is propulsive. As the foot transitions from stance to propulsion, the fulcrum moves medially from between the first and second metatarsals in line with the forward direction of gait. This shift places more stress on the first metatarsal and hallux, which have adapted with increased size and stability.[1,4]

CAUSES OF DYSFUNCTION IN THE MODERN HUMAN FOOT

Foot balance depends on both the architectural structure of the bones and ligaments as well as postural strength afforded by the muscles. A deficit of either leads to an unbalanced foot. Mechanical stresses and strains are the underlying causes of accumulative trauma. The accumulative trauma caused by uneven weight distribution because of faulty mechanics is the primary source of foot pathology.[1–3,6–8] The two parts of the foot most affected are the medial longitudinal arch and the metatarsals. The mechanical faults are compounded by repetitive stresses that can eventually result in the collapse or breakdown of the structure as a whole. Smaller, localized defects in one part of the foot can have a deleterious effect on the whole foot. If the foot has not fully evolved and these atavistic traits persist, problems can develop including common clinical presentations of hallux valgus, hallux limitus, lesser metatarsal overload, plantar fasciitis, midfoot arthrosis, and posterior tibial tendon dysfunction[6,7,9] (Fig. 5).

The modern human foot has evolved into a rigid structure with a much larger calcaneus and a medial longitudinal arch. The first ray has become dominant in size and parallel to the longitudinal axis of the foot. It has become a more efficient foundation for bipedal gait and propulsion.[1] Although it has retained muscles that were designed for grasping, they are now eccentrically loaded to stabilize the forefoot during midstance and push off. Moreover, in order to attain true upright posture, the posterior leg muscles had to elongate to allow the heel to bear weight. Similarly, the hindfoot has adapted to prevent the inward deflection of weight by raising the sustentaculum tali and creating a parallel talus and metatarsal axis.[1]

The evolution of the first ray is of particular interest because this is one of the main arguments anthropologists and evolutionary biologists have to connect the link between ape and man. By enlarging and elongating, the first ray acts as the fulcrum for improved leverage and as a buttress against the inward concentration of body weight. In comparing surfaces of the first metatarsocuneiform joint of lower primates and man, there is a progressive decrease in medial angulation, supporting the evidence that the modern human foot no longer has a divergent first metatarsal.[1–3] Through his observations and analyses, Morton attributed most foot pathology as a consequence of residual atavistic traits. Feet that still retain characteristics of an earlier state in evolution are less equipped to withstand ground reactive forces, thus resulting in dysfunction and pain. He determined that most foot cases represented accumulative trauma resulting from uneven weight distribution and faulty movement of stresses through the foot. Specifically, he identified equinus, first ray insufficiency, and a long second metatarsal as the 3 primary causes of foot pathologic condition.[1–3]

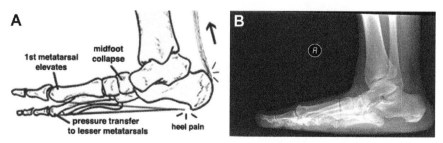

Fig. 5. (A, B) Equinus and first ray instability can affect the lesser metatarsals, midfoot, and medial longitudinal arch with myriad clinical presentations. (Photo courtesy of Christine Dobrowolski, DPM)

Morton observed 3 common atavistic traits that are responsible for the majority of foot problems.

1. Gastrocnemius equinus
2. Insufficient first ray
3. Relatively long second metatarsal

Dysfunction of the foot originates from an uneven distribution of weight where one portion is unable to compensate for the lack of work another portion should be carrying. Through a series of observational studies, Morton uncovered a common finding of a short or dorsally hypermobile first metatarsal segment. This was identified as the main culprit in foot dysfunction.[1–3] If the first metatarsal does not bear its fair share of weight and function, it gets transferred to the adjacent, relatively long second metatarsal. It is unable to provide a buttress to resist the inward deflection of body weight, and the persistent overpronation places undue strain on the muscles of the posteromedial ankle.[1–3,6–8] He found that these often occurred simultaneously. Impairment of the medial soft tissue restraints to pronation from failure of the medial longitudinal arch causes an array of symptoms and dysfunction. The stress of weight-bearing in a poorly designed foot with these structural deficits is repetitive. Most of the time, the structural deficits are not recognized until symptoms appear. As long as the unbalanced foot can tolerate the increased stress without failing, function is not affected. However, if the foot cannot withstand the stress then fatigue and failure ensue resulting in pain and inflammation. In a properly balanced foot, the first and second metatarsal heads equally share the fulcrum of the foot's leverage action.[7,10] In a foot with an insufficient first metatarsal, the fulcrum moves to the second metatarsal head, and sometimes the third[6,7,11,12] (**Fig. 6**). Excessive pressure under the second metatarsal head can cause a variety of symptoms including pain, callus, synovitis, second metatarsophalangeal joint (MTPJ) instability and subluxation, plantar plate tears, and stress

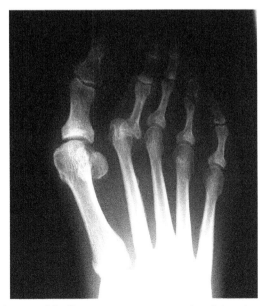

Fig. 6. A short or hypermobile first ray can cause second metatarsal overload, here manifested as subluxation of the second MTPJ.

fractures. The second and sometimes third metatarsophalangeal and tarsometatarsal joints can become inflamed, presenting as effusion, synovitis, and chronic traumatic arthrosis. The second metatarsal shaft often responds by developing a thicker cortical wall to counteract fatigue and fracture.[3,6,7] Morton emphasized that these should not be considered independent, incidental findings but rather classic signals of foot dysfunction.[1]

The lack of a first metatarsal buttress also affects the hindfoot. If the first ray cannot halt pronation because it is short or hypermobile, not rigid or supportive, then the strain on the medial border of the foot causes the sustentaculum tali to revert to its pre-human obliquity allowing the talus to fall plantarly and medially, accentuating the pronation of the foot as a whole (**Fig. 7**). Because the trochlear surface of the talus maintains a press fit position in the tibiotalar joint, the lower leg accommodates this deformity by internally rotating. The hip compensates by externally rotating, thus exaggerating the abducted position of the foot relative to the leg. The foot loses its effectiveness as a propulsive lever and the supinatory muscles of the hindfoot lose their mechanical advantage and become strained in their attempt to support a structurally unbalanced foot.[1,3,4] Morton supposed that the peroneals consequently spasm and overpower the medial supinators but recent evidence suggests otherwise. Electromyography (EMG) studies have shown that in patients with pronated feet, there is actually decreased activity in the peroneals, and increased activity in the tibialis posterior (PT), flexor digitorum longus (FDL), and flexor hallucis longus (FHL) muscles because they try harder to counteract the forces contributing to arch collapse.[13] If the majority of compensation is taken by the second metatarsal, then symptoms associated with metatarsalgia develop. If the stress is primarily absorbed by the medial soft tissue restraints, then symptoms associated with PTTD, hallux limitus, hallux valgus, and midfoot arthrosis develop. Morton knew that muscle weakness is not the predominant cause of structural deformity. Rather, it is caused by a hereditary defect in the bony architecture of the foot. The strain of the soft tissues is secondary. The attempt of the supinatory muscles to stabilize a structurally unbalanced foundation results in their failure if the degree of physical activity exceeds their ability to support the deficit.[1]

Subotnick postulated that "Equinus is the greatest symptom producer in the human foot."[14] Rush described the Achilles as a class II lever that creates a bending moment through the midfoot.[15] The medial column maintains a stable lever between the fulcrum of the forefoot and the primary input of the Achilles.[15] He coined the term "talar equinus" to highlight the existence of equinus on plain weight-bearing x-rays. In midstance of gait, as the swing leg aligns with the standing foot, a tight calf muscle

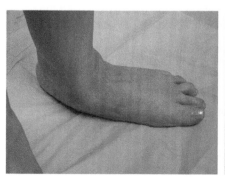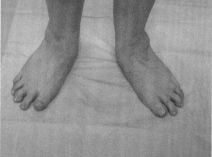

Fig. 7. If the first ray does not provide a buttress against pronation, it is unable to resist collapse of the medial longitudinal arch.

transmits stress to the talus, which compensates by providing a premature heel lift. Alternatively, the foot could gain the necessary amount of dorsiflexion from more distal joints but at the cost of stressing joints not designed to submit to a bending moment, resulting in midfoot arthrosis and stress fractures. These midfoot joints are designed to lock and provide rigidity to the beam as the foot propels forward. Structural rigidity is paramount to leverage.[1] This need for more dorsiflexion than the ankle can provide increases strain on the medial longitudinal arch similar to the effects of an insufficient first ray that provides no buttress. This is corroborated by Christensen's contemporary studies in the laboratory analyzing the effects of equinus on cadaveric feet.[9,16,17] Morton observed that shortening of the calf muscle is a primary cause of foot strain because it directly acts on the medial longitudinal arch.[1] Johnson and Christensen showed how equinus causes a bending moment in the midfoot, effectively flattening the arch and dampening the effects of peroneus longus to stabilize the first ray.[9,16]

TREATMENT

Uneven distribution of weight due to equinus and an insufficient first ray is the overarching theme in understanding Morton's conclusions regarding the link between faulty foot posture and disability. Identifying structural faults that are the primary cause of foot dysfunction is paramount to offering a treatment plan. The importance of treating the cause is as critical today as it was in Morton's time. A malaligned foot does not become symptomatic until it can no longer withstand the stresses exerted on it. Concentrated repetitive stress of the supporting tissues (bone, ligament, and tendon) will at first present as an acute inflammatory strain and later as chronic arthrosis and morphological changes. Many feet with poor postural architecture are painless as long as the stresses placed on them do not cross the threshold for pain.

There are two general phases of treatment. The first and more urgent is to reduce the symptoms. The acute inflammation needs to subside before the longer term goal of fixing the underlying mechanical disturbance can be achieved. Rest, ice, anti-inflammatory medication, and most importantly offloading the foot to allow the injured tissue time to heal are first steps. The symptoms will not resolve if constant, repetitive microtrauma of the tissues is not abated. Then, the mechanical faults that are the causes of the symptoms can be addressed in the second phase of treatment.

CONSERVATIVE TREATMENT

Structural and functional deficits associated with Morton's foot are manifested in a myriad of symptoms including Achilles problems, flatfoot deformity, arthrosis, first ray pathology, central metatarsalgia, and clawing of the toes. Addressing the cause of equinus and first ray insufficiency is critical in alleviating pain and dysfunction.

> "Analysis of foot balance discloses very clearly that the first metatarsal segment is the most important element of medial stability in the foot. That being the case, it is the part that must inevitably be affected when foot balance is impaired"
> —Dudley Morton, 1935.[1]

To address equinus, stretching of the calf muscles is important but, independently, it is not enough. A shoe with a slight heel elevation to effectively bring the ground to the heel, offloads the forefoot as well as mitigating pronation. Without a heel lift, the foot would need to compensate in order to allow the heel to contact the ground. This compensation takes the form of overpronation to gain the necessary dorsiflexion distal to the ankle. In some instances, the foot does not compensate, and instead, results in forefoot overload and early heel lift in gait. Applying a heel lift allows for more even

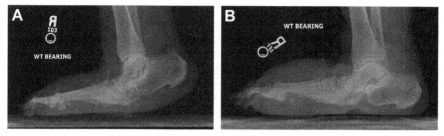

Fig. 8. (*A, B*) An exaggerated example of the effects of isolated tendo-Achilles lengthening on the medial longitudinal arch (*A*) preop and (*B*) postop.

distribution between the heel and forefoot. (new paragraph here)To address first ray dysfunction and lesser metatarsal overload, the midsole of the shoe must be stiff to support the medial column. Morton's understanding of biomechanics is evident in the way he describes supinatus. In response to overpronation, the supinators elevate the first ray to try to compensate for the medial deflection of body weight. Supinatus is essentially the result of the first ray bottoming out at its most dorsal excursion during pronation, and therefore in a position of elevatus when the hindfoot is aligned in neutral. A rigid foot orthosis not only redistributes the pressure away from the

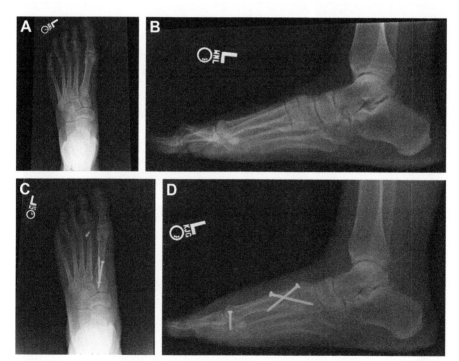

Fig. 9. Preoperative images of second metatarsal overload because of first ray instability, a relatively long second metatarsal, and gastrocnemius equinus (*A*) and (*B*). Correction of the deformity with gastrocnemius recession to address the equinus component, arthrodesis of the first tarsometatarsal joint to address the instability of the first ray, shortening of the second metatarsal with second MTPJ soft tissue balancing to address the local pathology (*C*) and (*D*).

metatarsal heads by increasing contact in the arch but also helps provide a retaining wall for the first ray supinatus. Adding a metatarsal pad immediately proximal to the second metatarsal head can exaggerate the offloading of the metatarsal. A stiff, supportive shoe with heel elevation to match the degree of equinus, combined with a rigid orthotic, helps resist overpronation and thus addresses symptoms associated with medial longitudinal arch collapse.

SURGICAL TREATMENT

Paul Lapidus is often credited with applying Morton's observations to surgical reconstruction of the foot.[18] Sigvard T. Hansen studied Morton's findings and applied Association of osteosynthesis (AO) principles of internal fixation to offer a more sophisticated surgical reconstruction. He espoused gastrocnemius lengthening and arthrodesis of the first tarsometatarsal joint as fundamental to addressing faulty foot mechanics and correcting pain and dysfunction. He described overpronation as dorsolateral peritalar subluxation because of equinus and medical column instability.[7,19] Jeff Christensen's seminal research in the Northwest Podiatric Foundation laboratory corroborated Morton's observations and supported Hansen's approach to surgically addressing these atavistic traits.[9,17] Surgical treatment is indicated

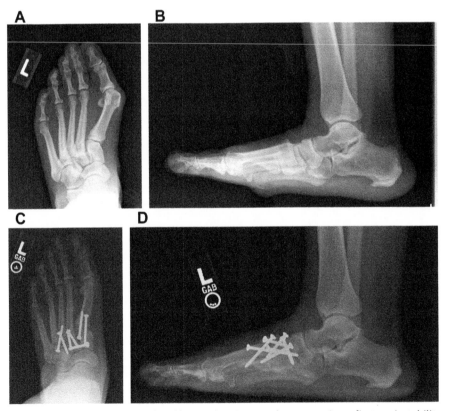

Fig. 10. Preoperative images of midfoot arthrosis secondary to equinus, first ray instability, and met adductus (*A*) and (*B*). Arthrodesis of the nonessential flat Roman arch pivot joints addresses the etiology and effects of equinus and first ray instability without sacrificing mobility or function (*C*) and (*D*).

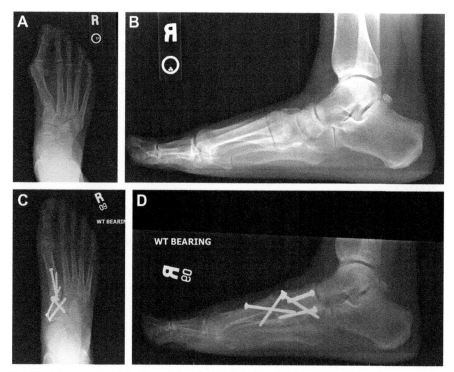

Fig. 11. Adult acquired flatfoot deformity with hallux valgus exhibiting Morton's observations of talar equinus, depression and obliquity of the sustentaculum tali, and a lack of a medial column buttress (A) and (B). Stabilization of the medial column via arthrodesis of the first tarsometatarsal and naviculocuneiform joints combined with gastrocnemius recession restores medial column stability and raises the sustentaculum tali as evidenced by realignment of the talar–first metatarsal axis (C) and (D).

when conservative treatment fails to adequately alleviate pain and dysfunction. The goals are the same. Lengthening of the gastrocsoleus complex and stabilization with realignment of the first ray should be considered critical components of the overall reconstruction of the foot (**Fig. 8**). Shortening of the second metatarsal to reestablish a normal metatarsal parabola is indicated if the metatarsal is abnormally long and symptomatic (**Fig. 9**). The medial longitudinal arch should be converted to a rigid lever to resist the shear forces and bending moment across it. This is accomplished by stabilizing what Hansen described as the nonessential joints of the "Roman arch."[7] These pivot joints are not supposed to move much. Fixing an unstable first ray by fusing the stressed joints in the medial arch improves its function as a propulsive lever (**Fig. 10**). It also provides a supinatory thrust on the hindfoot.[11,20] The talus is better aligned as its plantar medially directed load is resisted by a raised sustentaculum tali. Arthrodesis of the first tarsometatarsal joint as well as the naviculocuneiform joint has been shown to raise the medial longitudinal arch and realign the talar-first metatarsal axis (**Fig. 11**).[15,20]

SUMMARY

The foot has evolved into an efficient propulsive lever used for locomotion in a fully upright human; however, remnants of an earlier stage in its development remain and are responsible for the majority of foot problems patients develop. To alleviate pain and dysfunction in these patients, Hansen, Christensen, and others have demonstrated the importance of correcting equinus and first ray insufficiency. Lengthening of the gastrocnemius to offload the arch and forefoot, and stabilization of the medial column to provide a stable tripod arm to counter the upward shear force through the first metatarsal, are considered essential components of fixing an unstable, unbalanced foot.[7,9,11,12,15–17,19,21–23]

DISCLOSURES

The author has nothing to disclose.

REFERENCES

1. Morton DJ. The human foot: its evolution, physiology and functional disorders. Morninside Heights, New York: Coumbia University Press; 1935.
2. Morton DJ. Metatarsus atavicus: the identification of a distinctive type of foot disorder. J Bone Joint Surg Am 1927;9:531–44.
3. Morton DJ. Hypermobility of the first metatarsal bone. J Bone Joint Surg Am 1928; 10:187–96.
4. Morton DJ, Fuller DD. Human locomotion and body form: a study of gravity and man. 1st edition. Baltimore: Williams & Wilkins Company; 1952.
5. Keith A. Hunterian lectures on man's posture: its evolution and disorders. Br Med J 1923;1(3251):669–72.
6. Christensen JC, Jennings MM. Normal and abnormal function of the first ray. Clin Podiatr Med Surg 2009;26(3):355–71.
7. Hansen ST Jr. Functional reconstruction of the foot and ankle. Philadelphia: Lippincott Williams and Wilkin; 2000.
8. Hansen ST Jr. Introduction: the first metatarsal: its importance in the human foot. Clin Podiatr Med Surg 2009;26(3):351–4.
9. Johnson CH, Christensen JC. Biomechanics of the first ray. Part I. The effects of peroneus longus function: a three-dimensional kinematic study on a cadaver model. J Foot Ankle Surg 1999;38(5):313–21.
10. Stokes IA, Hutton WC, Stott JR. Forces acting on the metatarsals during normal walking. J Anat 1979;129(Pt 3):579–90.
11. King CM, Hamilton GA, Ford LA. Effects of the Lapidus arthrodesis and chevron bunionectomy on plantar forefoot pressures. J Foot Ankle Surg 2014;53(4):415–9.
12. Blitz NM. The versatility of the lapidus arthrodesis. Clin Podiatr Med Surg 2009; 26(3):427–41.
13. Murley GS, Landorf KB, Menz HB, et al. Effect of foot posture, foot orthoses and footwear on lower limb muscle activity during walking and running: a systematic review. Gait Posture 2009;29(2):172–87.
14. Subotnick SI. Equinus deformity as it affects the forefoot. J Am Podiatry Assoc 1971;61(11):423–7.
15. Rush SM, Jordan T. Naviculocuneifrom arthrodesis for treatment of medial column instability associated with lateral peritalar subluxation. Clin Podiatr Med Surg 2009;(3):374–84.
16. Johnson CH, Christensen JC. Biomechanics of the first ray part V: the effect of equinus deformity. A 3-dimensional kinematic study on a cadaver model. J Foot Ankle Surg 2005;44(2):114–20.

17. Roling BA, Christensen JC, Johnson CH. Biomechanics of the first ray. Part IV: the effect of selected medial column arthrodeses. A three-dimensional kinematic analysis in a cadaver model. J Foot Ankle Surg 2002;41(5):278–85.
18. Lapidus PW. The author's bunion operation from 1931 to 1959. Clin Orthop 1960; 16:119–35.
19. Sangeorzan BJ, Hansen ST Jr. Modified Lapidus procedure for hallux valgus. Foot Ankle 1989;9(6):262–6.
20. Avino A, Patel S, Hamilton GA, et al. The effect of the Lapidus arthrodesis on the medial longitudinal arch: a radiographic review. J Foot Ankle Surg 2008;47(6): 510–4.
21. Hansen ST Jr. Hallux valgus surgery. Morton and Lapidus were right. Clin Podiatr Med Surg 1996;13(3):347–54.
22. Ray RG, Ching RP, Christensen JC, et al. Biomechanical analysis of the first metatarsocuneiform arthrodesis. J Foot Ankle Surg 1998;37(5):376–85.
23. Dujela MD, Langan T, Cottom JM, et al. Lapidus arthrodesis. Clin Podiatr Med Surg 2022;39(2):187–206.

The Lapidus Bunionectomy Revolution

Current Concepts and Considerations

Christy M. King, DPM, FACFAS[a,b,*],
Francesca M. Castellucci-Garza, DPM, FACFAS[c,d]

KEYWORDS

- Hallux valgus • Hypermobility • First ray instability • Planes of deformity
- Fixation options • Early weight-bearing

KEY POINTS

- The modified Lapidus bunionectomy is a powerful procedure to address the hallux valgus deformity that has evolved over the years into a reproducible method to tackle instability of the first ray in all three planes.
- The surgeon must strive for a multiplanar correction, addressing all three planes of deformity, to help avoid or reduce the potential complications associated with this procedure, including recurrence or nonunion.
- Various fixation constructs have been used for the modified Lapidus bunionectomy without a clear consensus on ideal fixation technique.
- Weight-bearing after the modified Lapidus procedure with various fixation techniques has been shown to yield good results.

INTRODUCTION

The modified Lapidus bunionectomy is a dynamic and powerful procedure that not only addresses the common triplanar deformity of hallux valgus (HV) but also provides stability to the medial column. Whether discussing indications for performing the modified Lapidus bunionectomy, investigating superior fixation constructs, or determining if early weight-bearing is acceptable, there are few procedures within the foot and ankle literature that have garnered as much debate over the decades. The goal of this article is to attempt to appreciate both the complexity of the HV deformity,

[a] Kaiser San Francisco Bay Area Foot & Ankle Residency Program, Kaiser Oakland Foundation Hospital, 275 MacArthur Boulevard, Clinic 17, Oakland, CA 94611, USA; [b] Foot & Ankle Surgery, Orthopedics and Podiatry Department, Kaiser Oakland, Oakland, CA, USA; [c] Kaiser San Francisco Bay Area Foot & Ankle Residency Program, Kaiser Oakland Foundation Hospital, Oakland, CA, USA; [d] Foot & Ankle Surgery, Orthopedics and Podiatry Department, Kaiser Antioch, 4501 Sand Creek Road, Antioch, CA 94531, USA
* Corresponding author. 275 MacArthur Blvd, Clinic 17, Oakland, CA 94611.
E-mail address: Christy.m.king@kp.org

Clin Podiatr Med Surg 41 (2024) 43–58
https://doi.org/10.1016/j.cpm.2023.06.002
podiatric.theclinics.com

recognize important features and considerations with the modified Lapidus bunionectomy, discuss literature concerning fixation options and postoperative early weight-bearing, and examine where we still need to focus as a profession to improve results for our patients with HV deformity.

HISTORY

Numerous techniques have been presented over the years to address the common HV deformity. Albrecht was the first to describe a first tarsometatarsal joint (TMJ) arthrodesis to address this common deformity.[1] Following this procedure, Truslow performed a wedge resection of the first metatarsal cuneiform joint to focus on what he termed metatarsus primus varus.[2] It was not until the 1930s that the namesake for the Lapidus bunionectomy first presented the now commonly used procedure. The original Lapidus bunionectomy consisted of arthrodesis of the first metatarsal-cuneiform joint, arthrodesis of the first metatarsal base to the second, exostectomy of the first metatarsal head, and soft tissue repositioning.[3,4] He performed this extensive operation with the use of catgut suture for fixation which may have contributed to its increased complication rate and poor early acceptance. He was revolutionary at the time in his thought that the deformity should be corrected at the apex and hypothesized that the hypermobility of the first metatarsal-cuneiform joint, an increased intermetatarsal angle (IMA), and oblique joint axis predisposed patients to the development of the condition. In the 1980s, Sangeorzan and Sigvard Hansen transformed the original Lapidus by using rigid internal crossed screw fixation and addressing mainly the first metatarsal-cuneiform joint.[5] Over the last 40 years, joint preparation techniques, fixation methods, use of grafts, and postoperative management continue to evolve with the ultimate goal of increasing patient satisfaction and decreasing complication rates.

CONSIDERATIONS: ANATOMY OF HALLUX VALGUS

To truly appreciate what is needed to fully address the HV deformity, it is important to understand how it can occur. The first ray plays an essential role in maintaining the medial longitudinal arch of the foot and provides stability through the windlass mechanism. There is a constant balance between the static and dynamic stabilizers of the first ray, and extrinsic forces can play additional roles. The true etiology of HV deformity may vary in terms of what structures fail and when in the progression; however, there is an amalgamation of breakdowns that can contribute to this common deformity. Perera and colleagues described the avalanche of malfunctions that can occur in the HV deformity with some additions by other researchers along the way.[6,7] This process included failure of the medial ligaments along the first metatarsal-phalangeal joint (MTPJ), allowing the first metatarsal to move medially, increasing the first IMA, and exposing the sesamoids which appear more lateral. The abductor hallucis weakens and can no longer resist rotation of the first ray. The first MTPJ capsule further weakens and contributes to elevation of the first ray. This malalignment promotes weakness of the peroneus longus and inhibits its ability to stabilize the first ray. The plantar fascia is further destabilized, contributing to the instability of the medial column. There are multiple soft tissue structures that can fail in a variety of ways to produce the HV deformity (**Fig. 1**).

TRIPLANE DEFORMITY

HV is a triplanar deformity, and it is important for us to appreciate how each of the planes contributes to the classic features and measurements that we use for bunion

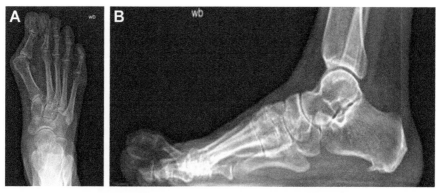

Fig. 1. Common hallux abduct valgus deformity with increased IMA, increased HA, valgus rotation of the hallux, and sub-second overload with hammertoe formation. There are multiple soft tissue structures that can fail in a variety of ways to produce the HV deformity (*A* and *B*).

deformities. From a radiographic perspective, the sagittal plane aspect of the deformity can be observed through a sag in the midfoot or elevation of the first ray on lateral radiographs (**Fig. 2**). From a clinical perspective, sagittal plane instability can be tested with the Hicks and dynamic Hicks testing. This test consists of holding the first ray at the first MTPJ with one hand and the lesser MTPJs in the other hand.[8,9] The evaluator then moves the first ray dorsal and plantar to determine the excursion present. The dynamic Hicks involves placing your hands in the same position while at the same time dorsiflexing the hallux to engage the windlass mechanism. Comparing these two tests helps to determine the level of first ray instability even in the presence of the stabilizing force of the plantar fascia. Shibuya and colleagues, in their systematic review, found statistically significant increased first ray motion in the sagittal plane in those with HV deformity as compared with those without.[10]

The transverse plane may be the simplest to identify with the classic measurements such as the IMA and hallux abductus angle on anterior posterior (AP) radiographs (**Fig. 3**). Myerson evaluated transverse plane instability clinically by strapping the forefoot with tape and then taking weight-bearing AP radiographs. If there was reduction of the first IMA with taping, then there is instability in the transverse plane.[11] Assessing the transverse plane instability even after initial first ray fixation can help to determine if a third screw or additional fixation is needed to stabilize the deformity.

The frontal plane is less straightforward to identify but has gained increasing attention. Radiographically, a sesamoid axial can help to evaluate both the valgus rotation of the first metatarsal along with its relationship to the sesamoid complex (**Fig. 4**). The "round sign" has also been described on AP radiographs in which valgus rotation first

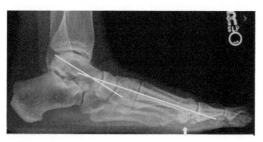

Fig. 2. Sagittal plane deformity.

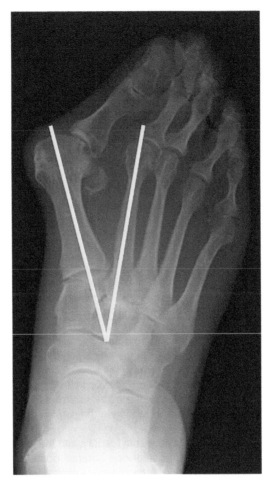

Fig. 3. Transverse plane deformity.

metatarsal head can be seen on the lateral aspect.[7] When this valgus rotation is corrected, the lateral aspect of the first metatarsal head should appear more linear. Appreciating this relationship is essential to ensuring the complete reduction of the deformity and helps to minimize recurrence. An accurate and reproducible measurement of pathologic frontal plane motion is difficult to capture. Cruz and colleagues described the pronatory rotation of about 15.36° in those patients with HV, whereas the normal feet in the study only had about 3.45°.[12] Ultimately, appreciating the deformity in all three planes and confirming realignment in each plane are necessary for the success of the procedure.

INDICATIONS

There are various indications for the modified Lapidus bunionectomy in the treatment of the HV deformity. Classically, the modified Lapidus bunionectomy has been used to address moderate to severe hallux abducto valgus, metatarsus primus varus, larger IMA (usually over 15°), hypermobility of the first ray, pain or callus sub-second metatarsal indicating lesser ray overload, arthrosis of the first or second metatarsal cuneiform

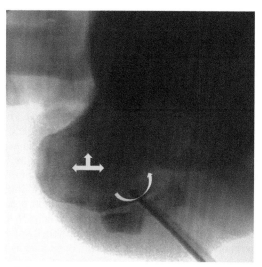

Fig. 4. Frontal plane deformity.

joint (**Fig. 5**), and recurrent HV. It can also be used to address medial column instability in addition to other pes planus procedures.

CONTROVERSIES: HYPERMOBILITY OR INSTABILITY OF THE FIRST RAY

Hypermobility of the first ray is an important driving motive for the utilization of the Lapidus bunionectomy; however, it is a controversial topic that can be difficult to define and hard to consistently quantify, contributing to the hesitation in acceptance. The hypermobility of the first ray in the case of HV should not be confused with hypermobile conditions such as Ehlers Danlos and Marfan , and it can be described in various ways including instability or lack of stiffness of the first ray. The lack of consistent measurements and variation in pathology makes it difficult to fully comprehend; however, it can play a significant role in the HV deformity.

Morton was the first to mention hypermobility in the 1920s, but it was not until Root in the 1977 was the first to define it as, "movement of the first metatarsal head above

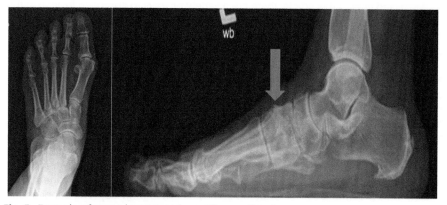

Fig. 5. Example of second metatarsal cuneiform arthrosis.

and below the transverse plane of the dorsiflexed lesser metatarsal heads."[3,8,13,14] In a series of articles highlighting the biomechanics of the first ray, Rush and colleagues described it as, "the excessive dorsal excursion with a soft endpoint."[15] Radiographically, we can see instability of the first ray with plantar gapping, sag in the midfoot, or elevated first ray. Clinically, we can observe hypermobility of the first ray with subsecond pain or callus or lateral foot overload as the first ray is not performing its role sufficiently.

Many have attempted to measure and quantify the deformity; however, there has been a lack of consistent results. Root quantified the hypermobility as moving the first metatarsal head 5 mm above and 5 mm below the transverse plane of the lesser metatarsal heads.[8] Klaue used a device to quantify hypermobility as 8 mm.[16] Following these studies, various others used degree of motion instead of millimeters. In those studies, the sagittal plane motion ranged from 10.5° to 14° in those with HV versus around 10.3° to 10.8° for the normal feet in the comparison group.[17-19] The Hicks and dynamic Hicks testing has also been used and was described in the previous section.[9] In an article discussing the complexities of hypermobility of the first ray, Roukis and colleagues recommended measuring the amount of excursion by placing the subtalar joint and ankle joint in neutral position, stabilizing the 2 to 5 metatarsals, and dorsiflexing the hallux at the same time.[9] Some argue that the difficulty defining and quantifying instability of the first should negate its use as a tool to direct procedure selection; however, it is important to at least consider its role in HV.

For others, its existence is clouded by the idea of whether it is truly a cause or an effect of HV. In a cadaver study by Rush and colleagues, he performed a proximal osteotomy, reducing the IMA to 5°, measured the motion of the first MTPJ in closed kinetic chain model, and he was able to reduce abnormal plantarflexion motion of the first MTPJ by 26%.[15] These results support the idea that by simply realigning the IMA, the windlass mechanism is placed on tension and is more efficient at supporting the first ray. In another cadaver study by Coughlin and colleagues, researchers performed a proximal crescentic osteotomy and reduced the mean sagittal range of motion from 11 to 5.22 mm. He concluded that the abnormal first ray motion developed secondary to the angular deformity.[20] These findings further muddle the ultimate understanding of hypermobility of the first ray, yet it is an important feature of the HV deformity to appreciate and consider.

THE MODIFIED LAPIDUS BUNIONECTOMY TECHNIQUE

As discussed later in this article, there are a variety of ways to approach fixation of the modified Lapidus bunionectomy; however, we detail below the typical technique used within our facility with some variations based on surgeon preferences or patient characteristics. Initially, attention is directed to the first ray, where a curvilinear incision is made, exposing both the first MTPJ and first TMJ (**Fig. 6**A). The incision is then deepened through subcutaneous tissue, taking care that vital neurovascular structures are carefully identified and retracted appropriately (**Fig. 6**B). The incision is carried down to the level of the first MTPJ capsule, where a linear capsulotomy is performed, exposing the first metatarsal head. Then, attention is directed to the first interspace, where a standard lateral release is performed, releasing both the sesamoid ligament and the conjoined tendon (**Fig. 6**C). There may be times that the sesamoid complex does not need to be released. Attention is directed to the first TMJ, where a transverse arthrotomy is performed. The joint is prepared for fusion, resecting all cartilage appropriately with a combination of osteotomes and curettes (**Fig. 6**D). The subchondral plate is fenestrated using a 2.0- to 2.5-mm drill bit or kirschner wire (k-wire) and fish-

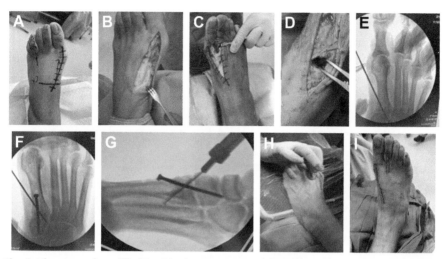

Fig. 6. The steps of modified Lapidus bunionectomy. (*A*) Incision planning. (*B*) Dissection to avoid the nerve, (*C*) Lateral capsulotomy and sesamoid release, (*D*) Cartilage removal at the first metatarsal-cuneiform joint (MCJ), (*E*) Temporary pinning of the first MCJ, (*F*) First screw placement from the dorsal distal first metatarsal to the plantar proximal medial cuneiform, (*G*) Second screw placement from the proximal dorsal medial cuneiform to the distal plantar first metatarsal base, (*H*) Stressing first interspace for residual transverse plane instability, (*I*) After skin closure.

scaled with an osteotome. The first metatarsal is then translated laterally to parallel the second metatarsal in both the sagittal and transverse plane and rotated as needed relocate the sesamoids into appropriate position. It is temporarily fixated with a k-wire in the corrected position (**Fig. 6**E). Fixation is typically achieved with two 3.5-mm cortical screws that are crossed and stacked. The screw directed from distal dorsal first metatarsal to proximal plantar medial cuneiform is placed first (**Fig. 6**F) followed by the second screw, directed from dorsal proximal medial cuneiform to distal plantar first metatarsal (**Fig. 6**G). For the final steps, the prominent medial eminence is resected using a rongeur, saw, or burr, if necessary. The distal capsule is then addressed if correction is needed at the first MTPJ. After stabilizing the capsule, the transverse plane is then tested for residual instability by attempting to create diastasis of the first interspace under fluoroscopy (**Figs. 6**H, **Fig. 7**). If residual instability is noted, a third point of fixation, typically from the medial cuneiform to the intermediate cuneiform, is inserted; however, other orientations can be performed. Intraoperative fluoroscopy is then used to assess screw position and realignment of the first ray in all three planes (**Fig. 6**I).

In some cases, the instability and valgus rotation in the frontal plane needs to be tackled before insertion of the two crossed screws. Some surgeons check the relationship between the sesamoids and the crista before surgery with a weight-bearing sesamoid axial radiograph, whereas others check a sesamoid axial intraoperatively before incision with simulated weight-bearing examination (**Fig. 8**). If the sesamoids rest with the first metatarsal head and crista, then the first metatarsal can be rotated into appropriate alignment without a sesamoid release (**Fig. 8**A). The reduction of the round sign can be appreciated on intraoperative fluoroscopy. If the sesamoids are in a more valgus position in relation to the crista, a sesamoid axial can help to appreciate their relationship (**Fig. 8**B and C) To help rotate the first metatarsal, a Kirschner wire is

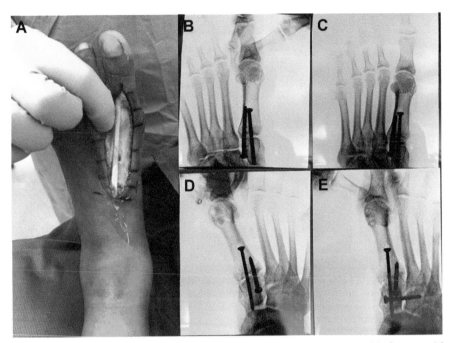

Fig. 7. Testing for residual (*A*) transverse plane instability. (*B* and *C*) shows stable first ray with testing which did not require a third point of fixation as compared to **Fig. 7** (*D* and *E*) which revealed residual instability, requiring third point of fixation between the cunieforms.

placed from dorsal to plantar and then rotated until the round sign has disappeared and the sesamoids are in appropriate alignment with the first metatarsal head (**Fig. 9**).

CONTROVERSIES AND CONSIDERATIONS: FIXATION CONSTRUCT AND WEIGHT-BEARING PROTOCOLS

Since the original Lapidus procedure, there have been multiple modifications in technique, fixation constructs, and utilization of an early weight-bearing postoperative protocol (**Fig. 10**). When attempting to determine a superior construct with the best outcomes, complication rates, primarily nonunion, and recurrence rates are important to consider (**Table 1**). In addition, hardware removal rates can also contribute to the

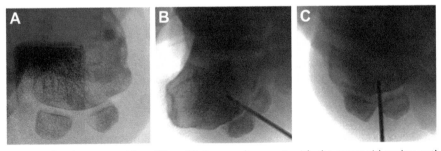

Fig. 8. Evaluating sesamoid position. (*A*) Proper alignment with the sesamoid underneath the first metatarsal head and between the crista, (*B*) First metatarsal head in overall proper alignment with valgus position of the sesamoids. (*C*) After reduction of the first metatarsal and sesamoids with modified Lapidus bunionectomy.

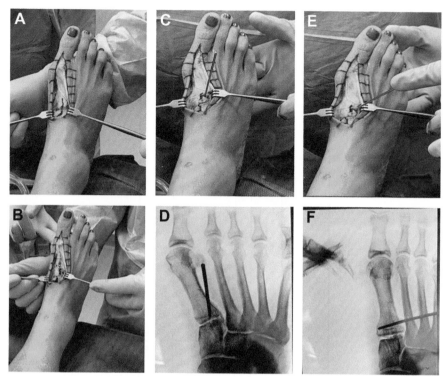

Fig. 9. Addressing frontal plane instability. (*A*) Prior to HV reduction. (*B*) Post reduction/rotation and screw stabilization, (*C*) Example of K-wire placed from dorsal to plantar in base of the first metatarsal, (*D*) Fluoroscopy images of initial K-wire position, (*E*) Clinical view of the rotation of the first ray with the K-wire, (*F*) Fluoroscopic evidence of rotation of the first ray and realignment of the sesamoids.

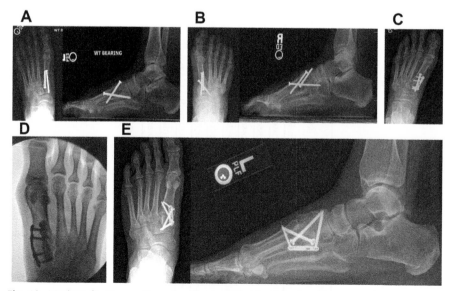

Fig. 10. Modern fixation options for the modified Lapidus bunionectomy. (*A*) Cross-screw fixation. (*B*) Cross-screw fixation with third screw. (*C*) Medial plate with dorsal interfragmentary screw. (*D*) Biplanar plate fixation. (*E*) Plantar plate.

Table 1
Fixation constructs with incidence of hardware removal and nonunion and weight-bearing status

Author, Year	Fixation	Weight-Bearing Status	HWR	Nonunion
Patel et al,[23] 2005	Crossed screws	Non-WB	5.3%	—
Blitz et al,[22] 2010	Crossed screws	Protected WB	0%	0%
King et al,[21] 2015	Crossed screws	Protected WB	2.2%	0%
Menke et al,[25] 2011	Medial plate with dorsal screw	Protected WB, 3–4 wk	0%	9.5%
Cottom et al,[26] 2013	Medial plate with plantar screw	Protected WB, 10 d	17%	2%
Saxena et al,[27] 2009	Dorsomedial plate with plantar screw	Protected WB, 4 wk	4.7%	0%
Sorenson et al,[38] 2009	Dorsomedial plate with screw	Protected WB, 2 wk	4.76%	9.5% (malunion)
Klos et al,[28] 2013	Plantar plate	Protected full WB	1.7%	1.69%
Liu et al,[33] 2022	Biplanar Plates	Protected WB, 8 d	5.1%	0.9%

Abbreviations: WB, weight-bearing; HWR, hardware removal.

perceived success and cost of the procedure. The different fixation constructs carry varying costs, and in the current health care climate, it is necessary to appreciate these potential differences (**Table 2**). In addition, the use of early weight-bearing and mobility without increasing the risks of failure or increased complications is valuable to consider. However, many of the current studies often tangle fixation construct and weight-bearing protocol, making it more difficult to determine the ideal construct and postoperative protocol. It is crucial to take in to consideration all of these topics when determining which fixation option is most beneficial in an individual surgeons' practice.

The original Lapidus bunionectomy was fixated with number 0 cat gut suture and there was noted to be high failure rates, likely in the setting of early weight-bearing without stable fixation.[3,4] Throughout the years, Kirschner wires, staples, external fixation, fusion rods, lag screws, and plates have all been documented fixation techniques. After a publication from Sangeorzan and Hansen in 1980s, the traditional cross-screw fixation became a more consistent fixation construct.[5] Current literature has evolved to show strong evidence that this cross-screw fixation in standard arbeitsgemeinschaft fur osteosynthesefragen (AO) technique has low nonunion rates and does permit early weightbearing.[21–24]

FIXATION OPTIONS: CROSS-SCREW FIXATION

Various studies have explored cross-screw fixation in the modified Lapidus bunionectomy. King and colleagues retrospectively reviewed 136 patients who underwent modified Lapidus arthrodesis with two cross screws and an early protected weight-bearing protocol. They found that early weight-bearing did not compromise deformity correction and their nonunion rate was less than 3%.[21] In addition, Blitz and colleagues used a two-screw construct with early protected weight-bearing and had a 100% union rate without any hardware complications.[22] Even before experimenting with early weight-bearing after cross-screw fixation, traditional non-weight-bearing protocols for the modified Lapidus procedure also showed good results.[23,24] Patel and colleagues reported on 227 cases of modified Lapidus arthrodesis performed with joint curettage, preservation of the subchondral plate, and cross-screw fixation with a 5.3% nonunion rate.[23]

Fixation Options: Plate and Screw Fixation

Following cross-screw fixation, various plate and screw combinations with different orientations have been described. A study by Menke and colleagues used a medial plate with dorsal screw and noted a 9.5% nonunion rate.[25] Early weight-bearing was initiated between 3 and 4 weeks, but the study found on average, patients began to fully bear weight with a pneumatic boot at 4.7 weeks (range of 3–7.5 weeks). A medial locking plate with a plantar interfragmentary screw was used by Cottom and Vora, and they noted a 2% rate of nonunion, but 17% of their patients required

Table 2 Hardware cost	
Hardware	**Cost**
Two 3.5/4.0 mm screws	$$
Locking plate + four locking screws	$$$-$$$$
Suture Endobutton	$$$
Biplanar plate	$$$$

hardware removal.[26] On average, the patients in this study population began to weight bear in a boot after 10 days. Saxena and colleagues used a dorsomedial locking plate and plantar screw with a 0% documented nonunion rate and compared with classic cross-screw fixation.[27] They permitted their patients with the plate fixation to bear weight in a boot at 4 weeks while continuing the cross-screw group with the classic non-weight-bearing protocol. Klos and colleagues used a plantar plate with a nonunion rate of 1.6%, supporting the importance of addressing the deformity on the side of tension.[28,29] Some advocate for the use of locking plates; however, other studies have shown that the use of plates does not consistently affect the rate of nonunion.[30–32] There is ongoing debate over the ideal fixation technique, even when a plate is used.

One of the most recent fixation techniques introduced, the biplanar plate fixation technique and utilization of cutting jig, custom reduction clamp. The most recent 2-year follow-up study by Liu and colleagues found positive patient outcome scores and radiographic results.[33] They also noted an overall complication rate of 13.7% with most related to hardware. Of those patients with hardware issues, 5.1% underwent hardware removal. In the study, there was overall nonunion rate of 0.9%.[34] With the current cost-conscious health care systems, it is important to consider the cost of this product.

FIXATION CONSTRUCT AND EARLY WEIGHT-BEARING PROTOCOL

A systematic review by Crowell and colleagues explored the nonunion rate after various fixation techniques and weight-bearing protocols.[35] Sixteen studies met their inclusion criteria and revealed an overall nonunion rate of 3.61%. They concluded that this was an acceptable nonunion rate to use the early weight-bearing protocol with various fixation constructs. More important than the fixation type used in any of these studies is the increased attention to reducing the deformity in all three planes and properly aligning the sesamoids and the first metatarsal head. Ultimately, there is no clear superior construct, and surgeons should use what they are more comfortable with and provides reliable results to address all three planes of deformity to maximize success for their patients. There is strong evidence to suggest that early weight-bearing for the modified Lapidus bunionectomy is a reasonable option in the setting of multiple fixation constructs including cross screw, interfragmentary screw and plate, or biplanar plate fixation. It is always important to review patient characteristics, as early weight-bearing may not be the best choice for all your patients. Ultimately, more studies are needed to isolate fixation construct and early weight-bearing protocols to determine the ultimate superior fixation and postoperative protocol.

FIXATION: ADDITIONAL TRANSVERSE PLANE INSTABILITY

After initial reduction and fixation of the HV deformity, it is important to evaluate if any residual transverse instability exists. A third point of fixation can be used to provide more stability to the construct by increasing load to failure, bending moment, and stiffness.[36] There can be various orientations of the third point of fixation used, including first to second metatarsal base, first metatarsal base to intermediate cuneiform, and medial to intermedial cuneiform (**Fig. 11**). A cadaver study by Feilmeier and colleagues noted that the greatest strength between those three constructs was found with the first to second metatarsal base screw, followed by the first metatarsal base to intermediate cuneiform screw, and last, with the medial to intermedial cuneiform screw.[37] A surgeon's utilization of the various third screw orientations may vary based on perceived stability needed. In contrast, the transverse plane instability can also be

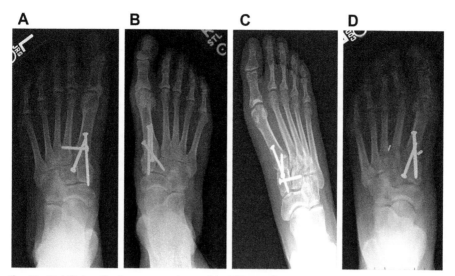

Fig. 11. Stabilizing the transverse plane with different fixation options. (*A*) From first metatarsal base to second metatarsal base. (*B*) From first metatarsal base to intermediate cuneiform. (*C*) From medial cuneiform to intermediate cuneiform. (*D*) Suture endobutton.

stabilized with a suture endobutton technique.[36] A study by King and colleagues evaluated a third screw, typically placed from first metatarsal base to second metatarsal base versus a suture endobutton for third point of fixation. Complication rates were similar between the two groups. Interestingly enough, sesamoiditis was higher in the third screw group, possibly suggesting that the utilization of this third screw orientation was more stiff, however this typically resolved around a year. There was a stress fracture in the suture endobutton group, and this is important to consider this potential complication when using this technique.

Although a third point of fixation may provide additional stability, it may also create a stress shielding environment that delays or inhibits boney consolidation, potentially contributing to a nonunion. Prissel and colleagues noted increased nonunion rate with the third screw construct; however, the position of the third screw was not documented.[32] We postulate that some patients may not tolerate when the medial column and central column are fixated together. Further research is needed to investigate whether the position of the third point of fixation can contribute to stability of the construct, decrease risk of nonunion, and be best tolerated by the patient.

SUMMARY

The HV deformity has plagued the human foot for centuries, and despite over a hundred different bunionectomy procedures described and multiple fixation options, there is no perfect procedure. It is essential to appreciate and address each patient's deformity in all three planes. There is no clear superior fixation technique, so it is necessary for each surgeon to feel comfortable with their selected technique to provide successful reduction and stabilization of the deformity while reducing chance of complications. Using an early weight-bearing protocol is supported in the literature, and the decision to use the protocol is also up each surgeon's comfort and patient characteristics.

CLINICS CARE POINTS

- It is essential to evaluate the deformity in all three planes and ensure they are addressed with the surgical correction.
- Multiple fixation options have been discussed; however, there is no clear superior construct. It is important for each individual surgeon to feel comfortable with their fixation technique to reduce the deformity and decrease the risk of complications whenever possible.
- The early weight-bearing protocol after multiple fixation techniques has been evaluated and noted to be successful. It is necessary for each surgeon to determine which fixation construct and patient population they feel most comfortable allowing early weight-bearing

DISCLOSURE

The authors have nothing to disclose.

REFERENCES

1. Albrecht GH. The pathology and treatment of hallux valgus. Russ Vrach 1911; 10(14):14–9.
2. Truslow W. Metatarsus primus varus or hallux valgus. J Bone Joint Surg Br 1925; 7:98.
3. Lapidus PW. The author's bunion operation from 1931 to 1959. Clin Orthop 1960; 16(12):119–35.
4. Lapidus PW. Operative correction of the metatarsal varus primus in hallux valgus. Surg Gynecol Obstet 1934;58:183–91.
5. Sangeorzan BJ, Hansen ST Jr. Modified Lapidus procedure for hallux valgus. Foot Ankle 1989;9(6):262–6.
6. Perera AM, Mason L, Stephens MM. The pathogenesis of hallux valgus. J Bone Joint Surg Am 2011;93(17):1650–61.
7. Dayton P, Feilmeier M, Kauwe M, et al. Relationship of frontal plane rotation of first metatarsal to proximal articular set angle and hallux alignment in patients undergoing tarsometatarsal arthrodesis for hallux abducto valgus: a case series and critical review of the literature. J Foot Ankle Surg 2013;52(3):348–54.
8. Root ML, Orien WP, Weed JH. Motion of the joints of the foot: the first ray. In: Root SA, editor. Clinical biomechanics. Volume II: normal and abnormal Function of the foot. Los Angeles: Clinical Biomechanics; 1977. p. 46–51.
9. Roukis TS, Landsman AS. Hypermobility of the first ray: a critical review of the literature. J Foot Ankle Surg 2003;42(6):377–90.
10. Shibuya N, Roukis TS, Jupiter DC. Mobility of the first ray in pateints with or without hallux valgus deformity: systematic review and meta-analysis. J Foot Ankle Surg 2017;56:1070–5.
11. Li S, Myerson MS. Evolution of thinking of the Lapidus procedure and fixation. Foot Ankle Clin N Am 2020;25:109–26.
12. Cruz EP, Wagner FV, Henning C, et al. Does hallux valgus exhibit a deformity inherent to the first metatarsal bone? J Foot Ankle Surg 2019;58(6):1210–4.
13. Morton DJ. Hypermobility of the first metatarsal bone: the interlinking factor between metatarsalgia and longitudinal arch strains. J Bone Joint Surg 1928; 10(3):187–96.
14. Morton DJ, editor. The human foot. Its Evolution, physiology, and Functional disorders. NY: Columbia University Press; 1935.

15. Rush SM, Christiansen JC, Johnson CH. Biomechanics of the first ray. Part II: metatarsus primus varus as a cause of hypermobility. A three-dimensional kinematic analysis in a cadaver model. J Foot Ankle Surg 2000;39(2):68–77.

16. Klaue K, Hansen ST, Masquelet AC. Clinical, quantitative assessment of first tarsometatarsal mobility in the sagittal plane and its relation to hallux valgus deformity. Foot Ankle Int 1994;15(1):9–13.

17. Prieskorn DW, Mann RA, Fritz G. Radiographic assessment of the second metatarsal: measure of first ray hypermobility. Foot Ankle Int 1996;17(6):331–3.

18. Lee KT, Young K. Measurement of first-ray mobility in normal vs. Hallux valgus patients. Foot Ankle Int 2001;22(12):960–4.

19. Faber FWM, Kleinrensink GJ, Verhoog MW, et al. Mobility of the first tarsometatarsal joint in relation to hallux valgus deformity: anatomical and biomechanical aspects. Foot Ankle 1999;20(10):651–6.

20. Coughlin MJ, Jones CP, Viladot R, et al. Hallux valgus and first ray mobility: a cadaveric study. Foot Ankle Int 2004;25(8):537–44.

21. King CM, Richey J, Patel S, et al. Modified Lapidus arthrodesis with crossed screw fixation: early weightbearing in 136 patients. J Foot Ankle Surg 2015;54: 69–75.

22. Blitz NM, Lee T, Williams K, et al. Early weightbearing after modified Lapidus arthrodesis: a multicenter review of 80 cases. J Foot Ankle Surg 2010;49:357–62.

23. Patel S, Ford LA, Etcheverry J, et al. Modified Lapidus arthrodesis: rate of non union in 227 cases. J Foot Ankle Surg 2004;43(1):37–42.

24. Kopp FJ, Patel MM, Levine DS, et al. The modified Lapidus procedure for hallux valgus: a clinical and radiographic analysis. Foot Anke Int 2005;26(11):913–7.

25. Menke CRD, McGlamry MC, Camasta CA. Lapidus arthrodesis with a single lag screw and a locking H-plate. J Foot Ankle Surg 2011;50(4):377–82.

26. Cottom JM, Vora AM. Fixation of Lapidus arthrodesis with a plantar interfragmentary screw and medial locking plate: a report of 88 cases. J Foot Ankle Surg 2013; 52(4):465–9.

27. Saxena A, Nguyen A, Nelsen E. Lapidus bunionectomy: early evaluation of crossed lag screws versus locking plate with plantar lag screw. J Foot Ankle Surg 2009;48(2):170–9.

28. Klos K, Wilde CH, Lange A, et al. Modified Lapidus arthrodesis with plantar plate and compression screw for treatment of hallux valgus with hypermobility of the first ray: a preliminary report. Foot Ankle Surg 2013;19(4):239–44.

29. Klos K, Gueorguiev B, Muckley T, et al. Stability of medial locking plate and compression screw versus two crossed screws for Lapidus arthrodesis. Foot Ankle Int 2010;31(2):158–63.

30. Barp EA, Erickson JG, Smith HL, et al. Evaluation of fixation techniques for metatarsocuneiform arthrodesis. J Foot Ankle Surg 2017;56(3):468–73.

31. Donnenwerth MP, Borkosky SL, Abicht BP, et al. Rate of nonunion after first metatarsal-cuneiform arthrodesis using joint curettage and two crossed compression screw fixation: a systematic review. J Foot Ankle Surg 2011;50:707–9.

32. Prissel MA, Hyer CF, Grambart ST, et al. A multicenter, retrospective study of early weightbearing for modified. Lapidus Arthrodesis 2016;55:226–9.

33. Liu GT, Chhabra A, Dayton MJ, et al. One- and two-year analysis of a five-year prospective multicenter study assessing radiographic and patient-reported outcomes following triplanar first tarsometatarsal arthrodesis with early weightbearing for symptomatic hallux valgus. J Foot Ankle Surg 2022. https://doi.org/10. 1053/j.jfas.2022.04.008. S1067-2516(22)00118-1.

34. Manchanda K, Chang A, Wallace B, et al. Short term radiographic and patient outcomes of a biplanar plating system for triplanar hallux valgus correction. J Foot Ankle Surg 2021;60:461–5.
35. Crowell A, Van JC, Meyr AJ. Early weightbearing after arthrodesis of the first metatarsal-medial cuneiform joint: a systematic review of the incidence of nonunion. J Foot Ankle Surg 2018;57(6):1204–6.
36. King CM, Doyle MD, Castellucci-Garza FM, et al. Addressing transverse plane instability in the modified Lapidus arthrodesis: a comparative study of screw versus suture and button fixation device technique. J Foot Ankle Surg 2022; 61(5):979–85.
37. Feilmeier M, Dayton P, Kauwe M, et al. Comparison of transverse and coronal plane stability at the first tarsal-metatarsal joint with multiple screw orientations. Foot Ankle Spec 2017;10(2):104–8.
38. Sorensen MD, Hyer CF, Berlet GC. Results of lapidus arthrodesis and locked plating with early weight bearing. Foot Ankle Spec 2009;2:227–33.

Early Functional Rehabilitation in Foot and Ankle Surgery

Sandeep Patel, DPM, FACFAS[a],*,
Shontal Behan Dionisopoulos, DPM, FACFAS[b],
Monte Jay Schmalhaus, DPM[c]

KEYWORDS

- Early weight bearing • Postoperative protocol • Lapidus bunionectomy
- First metatarsophalangeal joint arthrodesis • Ankle open reduction internal fixation

KEY POINTS

- Early weight bearing has been shown to be beneficial and safe in many postoperative protocols regarding foot and ankle surgery.
- Multiple systematic reviews have demonstrated that the various fixation techniques for first metatarsophalangeal joint arthrodesis result in similar union rates with early weight bearing.
- With a better understanding of technical principles, the modified Lapidus procedure has acceptable union rates with early weight bearing.
- There is a growing trend with early weight bearing and mobilization with ankle open reduction internal fixation with varying types of fractures and patient population.

INTRODUCTION

Postoperative management has always been considered a critical component in dictating surgical outcomes. The duration of immobilization and weight bearing status vary depending on the physician and surgery performed.

Historically, patients were nonweight bearing for a minimum of 6 weeks following elective and traumatic osseous procedures such as open reduction internal fixation (ORIF) of ankle fractures, arthrodesis of first tarsometatarsal (Lapidus), and first metatarsophalangeal joint arthrodesis.[1] These protocols are often implemented to reduce the incidence of complications such as nonunion, fracture displacement, loss of

[a] San Francisco Bay Area Foot and Ankle Residency, The Permanente Medical Group, Diablo Service Area, 1425 South Main Street, Walnut Creek, CA 94596, USA; [b] The Permanente Medical Group, Diablo Service Area, 1425 South Main Street, Walnut Creek, CA 94596, USA; [c] 104 East Hawthorne Street, Arlington Heights, IL 60004, USA
* Corresponding author.
E-mail address: sbpatel21@gmail.com

Clin Podiatr Med Surg 41 (2024) 59–71
https://doi.org/10.1016/j.cpm.2023.07.001
0891-8422/24/© 2023 Elsevier Inc. All rights reserved.

reduction, hardware failure, and wound complications.[2–6] However, patients may not have the capacity to remain nonweight bearing, and associated risks warrant consideration. Prolonged periods of nonweight bearing predispose the patient to risk of deep vein thrombosis (DVT), disuse osteopenia, cardiovascular complications, and generalized deconditioning.[1,2,7]

The decision to allow early weight bearing after foot and ankle surgery depends on the procedure, surgeon preference, and patient factors. Potential benefits of early weight bearing after foot and ankle surgery include prevention of deconditioning and atrophy, prevention of joint stiffness, and overall improvement in the patient's quality of life in activities of daily living during the perioperative period.

There has been a progression towards early weight bearing and rehabilitation in many areas of foot and ankle surgery. In addition to early weight bearing with osseous procedures, early rehabilitation protocols have gained significant popularity in the management of Achilles tendon ruptures. Numerous studies looking at surgical and nonsurgical management of Achilles tendon ruptures have shown benefits of early range of motion (ROM) and loading of the tendon in regards to improved outcomes.[8] Furthermore, improved fixation techniques for management of tendon pathology in the lower extremity and performing lateral ankle stabilization have also shown positive outcomes with early ROM and loading of the extremity.[9,10] These studies show the benefits of early loading on tissue healing and differentiation of collagen.

The authors' institution has contributed several articles reviewing the outcomes of early weight-bearing after operative treatment of foot and ankle conditions. In particular, the contributors have been reviewing the outcomes of first metatarsal phalangeal joint arthrodesis, the Lapidus bunionectomy, and open reduction internal fixation of ankle fractures.

FIRST METATARSOPHALANGEAL JOINT ARTHRODESIS

Arthrodesis of the metatarsophalangeal joint (MTPJ) is a reliable treatment option for addressing various conditions, including hallux rigidus, severe or recurrent hallux abductovalgus, and iatrogenic hallux varus. To achieve a successful fusion, it is crucial to properly prepare the joint, position it correctly, and use rigid internal fixation. Postoperative protocols for this procedure may range from immediate weight bearing in a postoperative shoe to nonweight bearing in a cast. Although some surgeons recommend delayed weight bearing to minimize the risk of hardware migration and nonunion, others advocate for early weight bearing with the advancement of rigid fixation techniques. This allows patients to walk on the operated foot almost immediately after surgery, preventing deconditioning and other risks associated with prolonged weight bearing (eg, muscular atrophy or thrombotic events)[11,12]

To promote postoperative stability, facilitate early weight bearing, and achieve successful union following first MTP fusion, it is essential to use rigid internal fixation. Surgeons often use multiple different fixation types, but the optimal method remains a topic of debate and varies significantly among practitioners. In a retrospective study of 132 patients, Hyer and colleagues[13] evaluated the outcomes of 4 different plate and/or screw constructs used to achieve fusion. They found that there was no significant difference in time to fusion or rate of fusion between static and locked plates, with or without a lag screw. The mean times to radiographic union and rate of fusion were as follows: static plate (59 days, 95% rate of fusion), static plate with lag screw (56 days, 86% rate of fusion), locked plate (66 days, 92% rate of fusion), and locked plate with lag screw (53 days, 96% rate of fusion). Mayer and colleagues[14] (2014) compared locking with nonlocking plates and found a significant difference in clinical healing, favoring the nonlocking plate, but no significant difference in time to radiographic union. They observed an overall 92% union rate in both groups. Many other studies have also reported on outcomes of early weight bearing after first metatarsophalangeal joint arthrodesis (**Table 1**).

Several systematic reviews have been performed to evaluate the effects of different types of fixation and early weight-bearing protocols on nonunion frequency. Crowell and colleagues[15] performed a review that analyzed 17 studies involving 898 feet. Their review included different types of fixation constructions and postoperative weight-bearing protocols used in first MTPJ arthrodesis. Of the 898 feet, 57 cases (6.35%) developed nonunion. Another systematic review of 16 studies involving 934 feet, by Füssenich and colleagues,[16] found the overall nonunion rate of 7.7% following different joint preparation types, joint fixation techniques, and postoperative weight-bearing protocols. A 5.1% nonunion rate was found following postoperative full weight bearing on a flat shoe versus 9.3% for full weight bearing on a heel weight-bearing shoe and 0% for a partial weight-bearing regimen. They also evaluated different fixation techniques and found a nonunion rate of 2.8% for joint fixation with a plate combined with a lag screw versus 6.5% for plate fixation, 11.1% for crossed-screw fixation, and 12.5% for a plate with a cross-plate compression screw. A systematic review performed by Roukis and colleagues examined union rate after first MTP fusion without early weight bearing and found it to be 5.4%, comparable to the previously mentioned studies that allowed for early weight bearingk. This supports that for certain patients, nonweight bearing after first MTP fusion is likely unnecessary and does not decrease the risk of nonunion.[17]

In a more recent study published out of the authors' institution, West and colleagues[18] retrospectively assessed the rate of radiographic union rates between crossed screws and dorsal plating in first MTPJ arthrodesis. There was an overall fusion rate of 93.5%, and there was no detectable difference in fusion rates at 12 weeks postoperatively within a heterogeneous population. They concluded, crossed screws and conventional plates are a reliable and inexpensive way to achieve first MTPJ arthrodesis (**Fig. 1**).

THE MODIFIED LAPIDUS BUNIONECTOMY

The Lapidus bunionectomy is a popular procedure to address bunion deformities. Historically, this procedure was often reserved for significant deformities with large intermetatarsal angles. However, the focus on triplanar correction in addressing medial column instability has emphasized the indications for the Lapidus bunionectomy.[19] In addition, the theoretical indication to address medial column instability and restore weight bearing through the first ray has been validated in clinical studies.[20,21] Along with this, improved fixation techniques and joint preparation have made this a more significant part of training, making the Lapidus bunionectomy more commonplace in the authors' practices. In addition, many surgeons had reservations regarding performing the surgery secondary to the technical demands and prolonged postoperative convalescence period. Of these, a prolonged course of nonweight bearing was often the recommended postoperative management.

The main reasoning for the prolonged nonweight bearing was a concern of high nonunion rates and complications.[22–26] However, with improved fixation and preparation techniques, those nonunion rates were shown to range between 2% to 10%.[22–27] The authors published their data in 2005, which, at the time, were the largest studies showing a nonunion rate of 5.3% when patients were kept nonweight bearing for a period of 6 weeks.[27] However, since that time, most literature has moved towards

Table 1
Summary of articles focusing on the outcome of early weight-bearing following arthrodesis of the first metatarsophalangeal joint

Authors	Patient Cohort	Length of Follow-Up	Weight-bearing Status	Immobilization	Outcomes
Zadik et al, 1960	N = 110	Minimum follow-up 4 weeks	Early weight bearing first week	Short-leg cast	5% nonunion rate
Mann et al, 1980	N = 41	Minimum follow-up 5 months	Early weight bearing first week	Surgical shoe	5% nonunion rate
Johansson et al, 1984	N = 60	Average 39 months	Early weight bearing first week	Short-leg cast	4% nonunion rate
Smith et al, 1992	N = 31	Minimum follow-up 12 months	Early weight bearing first week	Short-leg cast	3% nonunion rate
Niskanen et al, 1993	N = 39	Minimum follow-up 6 months	Early weight bearing first week	Wedge heel	18% nonunion rate
Sage et al, 1997	N = 12	Average 6.9 months	Early partial weight bearing first week	Surgical shoe, crutch/walker assistance	0% nonunion rate
Dayton et al, 2004	N = 43	Minimum follow-up 12 weeks	Immediate weight bearing on the heel or lateral foot	Surgical shoe	0% nonunion rate
Coughlin et al, 2005	N = 21	Minimum 24-month follow-up	Heel weight bearing at 10 days postoperatively	Surgical shoe	14% nonunion rate
Hyer et al, 2014	N = 116	Minimum follow-up 12 months	Weight bearing initiated within 10 postoperative days	Did not specify	9% nonunion rate
Storts and Camasta, 2016	N = 97	Minimum follow-up 12 months	Immediate weight bearing	Surgical shoe	3% nonunion rate
West et al,[18] 2022	N = 305 Dorsal plate 147 Crossed Screw 158	Minimum follow-up 12 months	Early weight bearing in dorsal plate group at 2 weeks	Did not specify	Screws 4.7% nonunion rate Plate group 6.5% nonunion rate Overall union rate similar regardless of fixation technique

It further includes weight-bearing status, method of immobilization, and results of union rate.

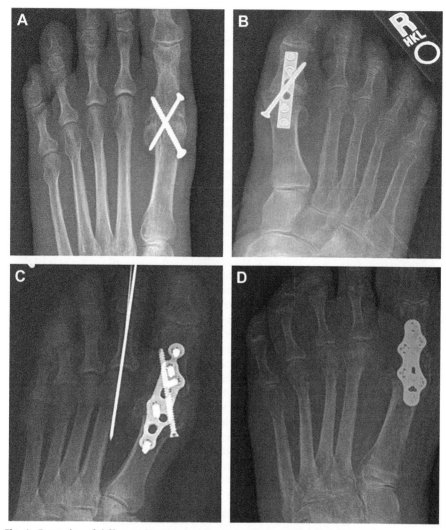

Fig. 1. Examples of different fixation constructs for first metatarsophalangeal joint arthrodesis. Crossed screws (*A*), screw and ¼ tubular plate (*B*), screw and anatomic plate (*C*), and anatomic plate alone (*D*). The authors' study along with review of the literature demonstrates that all constructs are suitable for early protected weight bearing.

early weight bearing. The authors feel there are several factors that contribute to this trend.

The influences can be simplified by looking at anatomical and biomechanical factors. The medial cuneiform has been shown to be a well-vascularized bone with vascular supply contribution from planter and dorsal branches.[28] Understanding the vascular anatomy is an important factor in understanding how to approach the joint without devascularization of the arthrodesis site. The authors prefer to do a transverse capsulotomy, thus maintaining the periosteum, and not violating the plantar branches to the medial cuneiform and the base of the first metatarsal. Furthermore, careful attention is placed in the joint preparation. The authors generally use the curettage technique but focus on removal of the subchondral plate. Schuberth and Christian demonstrated the importance of removing the subchondral plate when using the curettage technique.[29] They performed a histologic study on cadaveric models after removing the cartilage while maintaining the subchondral plate. They demonstrated a layer of calcified cartilage that covered more than 90% of the joint surface. It was suggested this layer of tissue may impede bone healing, and it is imperative to penetrate or remove this layer altogether. Although drilling or scaling may achieve this in part, it may still leave behind a high enough percentage of the surface area to result in a nonunion. The authors generally remove all of the subchondral bone to expose the underlying trabecular bone.

In addition to some of these anatomic considerations, there are likely several biomechanical factors that may contribute to early weight bearing. In evaluating the biomechanics of the medial column, it has been shown that the medial tarsometatarsal joint has the least amount of motion in the sagittal and frontal plane.[30] This, combined with the diabetic literature that shows significant offloading of the forefoot and midfoot with the use of controlled ankle motion walker or short leg cast,[31] provides confidence that the medical cuneiform is stress shielded with protected weight bearing. Finally, there are several biomechanical, cadaveric studies that have evaluated the various fixation techniques for the arthrodesis of the medial tarsometatarsal.[32–35] The authors' typical fixation involves 2 cross screws. Unlike the cadaveric studies that compare partially threaded cancellous screws, the authors make a point to purchase multiple cortices with larger bore cortical screws. The first group is inserted in standard lag fashion from the first metatarsal into the medial cuneiform with little attention in capturing the plantar medial aspect of the proximal aspect of the medial cuneiform. The second screws are inserted from the medial cuneiform towards the base of the first metatarsal. This is a positional screw. This construct captures at a minimum of 3 cortices, which theoretically improve the pullout strength (**Fig. 2**).

There are numerous clinical studies looking at the outcomes of the early weight-bearing after Lapidus bunionectomy (**Table 2**). The multicenter study by Prissel and colleagues[2] demonstrated no increased risk of nonunion in 367 patients undergoing the Lapidus procedure with early weight bearing compared to delayed weight bearing. This study evaluated varying methods of joint preparation and fixation, demonstrating safety in early weight bearing irrespective of technique. King and colleagues[3]

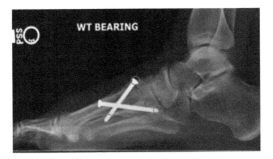

Fig. 2. Lateral projection of modified Lapidus fixation. This is an example of our crossed screw technique. The first screw is inserted in a standard lag technique with either a 3.5 or 4.0 mm cortical screw. It is directed from the midshaft of the first metatarsal to the plantar medial aspect of the medial cuneiform. The second screw is placed from the medial cuneiform aimed to the base of the first metatarsal. This is usually a 3.5 mm cortical screw placed in a positional fashion. This construct allows for purchase of 3 cortices to improve pull-out strength.

Table 2
Review of the literature reporting on the outcome of early weight bearing following modified Lapidus bunionectomy

Authors	Patient Cohort	Weight-bearing Status	Immobilization	Outcomes
King et al,[3] 2015	N = 136	Early WB within 8–21 days postoperatively	CAM Boot	Nonunion rate: 2.2%
Prissel et al,[2] 2016	N = 367	Early WB < 21 days Delayed WB > 21 days	CAM boot: 267 Cast: 90 Postoperative shoe: 10	Nonunion rate: 6.5% Early WB: 7.1% Delayed WB: 6.0%
Blitz et al, 2010	N = 80	WB at 2 weeks	CAM boot	Nonunion rate: 0%
Basile et al, 2010	N = 24	Immediate WB	CAM boot	Nonunion rate: 0%
Cottom et al,[32] 2013	N = 88	WB at 7–10 days	CAM boot	Nonunion rate: 2%
Ray et al, 2019	N = 62	WB at 2 weeks	CAM boot	Nonunion rate: 1.6%

Abbreviation: WB, weight-bearing

evaluated early weight bearing with traditional crossed screw fixation for modified Lapidus arthrodesis at the authors' institution. The authors reviewed 136 consecutive patients and found an overall nonunion rate of only 2.2%. This study demonstrated that patients could load their foot in a protected fashion at 2 weeks with a low number of complications, high union rate, and maintenance of deformity correction.

ANKLE FRACTURES

Traditionally, immobilization and nonweight bearing for more than 6 weeks has been the standard protocol for patients undergoing ORIF after ankle fracture. The purpose of this protocol was to minimize the risk of implant failure, delayed union, nonunion, loss of reduction, and fracture displacement. However, early weight bearing and ROM are now believed to offer several advantages in rehabilitation and return to function while minimizing complications such as muscle atrophy, disuse osteopenia, and joint stiffness.[5,36–39]

Early postoperative weight bearing after rotational ankle fractures is recommended after 2 weeks of surgery or until the incision has healed. This is because of an increased risk of wound healing complications with immediate postoperative weight bearing. While the increased risk of wound complications with immediate weight bearing did not reach statistical significance in multiple studies,[4,40–44] it can still be minimized by restricting protected weight bearing until the skin heals.

For most healthy patients with bimalleolar fractures, or equivalent injuries, weight bearing as tolerated within 2 weeks of surgical repair is widely accepted. Kaiser studies have been important in advancing the practice of early weight bearing after ankle repair. One of the earliest studies published in North America was performed in the authors' institution in 2012 by Starkweather and colleagues. They demonstrated that unstable unimalleolar and bimalleolar ankle fractures can be fully weight bearing in a short leg walking cast within 2 weeks of operative repair without risk of hardware failure, fracture displacement, or significantly greater risk of wound complications.[6] There are now several reports that have presented the benefits of early weight bearing and early ROM after ORIF in acute rotational ankle fractures without syndesmotic fixation, including improved ankle ROM.[4–7,36,43,45–47] These patients are generally allowed to weight bear as tolerated in a CAM boot and start early ROM and ultimately transition out of the boot once radiographic fracture healing is noted at 6 to 8 weeks.

Following the acceptance of early weight bearing in bimalleolar ankle fractures, trimalleolar ankle fractures and syndesmotic instability were investigated. In 2020, the authors' program reviewed the outcomes of early weight bearing in a cast following trans-syndesmotic screw fixation in rotational ankle fractures.[48] Trimalleolar ankle fractures were included in this study if the posterior malleolar fracture was not fixated. The study demonstrated that unstable ankle fractures with syndesmotic disruption can be fully weight bear without hardware failure, loss of reduction, or an increase in complications.

Again, the concern for early weight bearing following unstable ankle fixation was increased strain to fractures and hardware migration with cyclical loading to the operative limb. However, it is now appreciated that rotational forces are dampened by a walking cast, eliminating rotatory forces to the fibula. Furthermore, the lack of sagittal plane motion of the talus thwarts any burden to the fibula that develops with dorsiflexion past neutral, negating concerns of displacement or increased stress to implants.

The stability of the ankle following direct posterior malleolar fixation is the last element to consider in the investigation of early weight bearing in unstable rotational ankle fractures. Although clinical studies specifically investigating early weight bearing following direct posterior malleolar fixation are currently being conducted within Kaiser, studies have found that there is no posterior instability following posterior malleolar fracture repair.[49–52] The ankle has an instantaneous center of rotation where the poster malleolus can only be loaded with the ankle in plantar flexion.[53] Immobilizing the ankle in neutral with a short leg cast establishes talotibial contact pressures at the center of the tibial plafond.[53] Fitzpatrick and colleagues[50] found that after recreating a fracture line encompassing 50% of the posterior malleolus, the axial load is still placed anterior to the fracture line, supporting the notion that there is no inherent risk

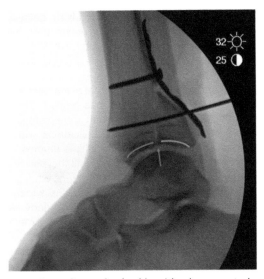

Fig. 3. Sagittal intraoperative radiograph of ankle with a large posterior malleolar fracture. The arrow depicts the fracture line. The weight-bearing surface of the ankle while dorsiflexed is anterior to the fracture line (*blue line*), showing the posterior half of the tibial plafond (*green line*) is not loaded with postoperative immobilization (cast).

Table 3
Summary of articles focusing on the outcomes of early weight bearing following ankle open reduction internal fixation

Authors	Patient Cohort	Length of Follow-up	Weight-bearing Status	Immobilization	Outcomes
Starkweather et al,[6] 2012	N = 126	Minimum of 42 days (average 171 days)	EWB within 15 days postoperatively	SLWC	Nonunion – 0%
Pyle et al, 2019	N = 31	Minimum 6 months	Average EWB 17.8 days	CAM boot	Nonunion – 0%
King et al,[52] 2020	N = 58	Minimum 12 months	EWB within 15 days postoperatively	SLWC	Nonunion – 0%
Passias et al, 2020	N = 95 EWB = 38 NWB = 57	Minimum 12 months	EWB average of 3.1 weeks	Did not say	Nonunion EWB = 0% Nonunion LWB = 4%
Park et al, 2021	N = 194 EWB = 95 NWB = 99	Minimum 12 months	EWB 2 weeks postoperatively	Removable walking cast	Return to preinjury activities faster in EWB– $P<.001$ Nonunion- 0%
Myers et al, 2021	N = 185 EWB = 47 LWB = 138		EWB within 3 weeks		Nonunion EWB = 2.1% LWB = 4.3%

It further includes weight-bearing status, immobilization methods, and results of union rate.
Abbreviations: EWB, early weight bearing; NWB, nonweight bearing; SLWC, short leg walking cast.

of fracture loading to cause displacement or hardware failure. In fact, multiple studies suggest this notion that with stable medial and lateral constraints, posterior subluxation will only occur in fractures larger than 40% of the tibial plafond[50,54–57] **(Fig. 3)**.

Lastly, variations in early mobilization after ankle ORIF must be considered in pathologic fractures and patients with a history of diabetes. Early ambulation may be beneficial for diabetic patients, as it can facilitate functional recovery and reduce the risk of cardiovascular complications.[40,46] Again, the authors' institution conducted one of the first studies on early weight-bearing outcomes after ankle fractures in diabetic patients. Although the literature has shown a higher complication rate in diabetic patients with ankle fractures, Bazarov and colleagues[47] demonstrated that early protected weight bearing can be safely practiced in a certain subset of diabetic patients with few known diabetic-related comorbidities **Table 3**.

SUMMARY

With the large database available at Kaiser Permanente, the authors have been fortunate to follow and evaluate the various postoperative protocols. Similar to numerous studies that have been performed looking at the benefits and outcomes of early weight bearing with some of the more common foot and ankle procedures, the authors' data also demonstrate the efficacy and safety of allowing early weight bearing in first MTPJ arthrodesis, modified Lapidus bunionectomy, and in many instances of open reduction internal fixation ankle fractures.

CLINICS CARE POINTS

- Regardless of fixation technique, early weight bearing is safe in first metatarsophalangeal joint arthrodesis
- With careful joint preparation and fixation techniques, the Lapidus bunionectomy can be allowed to weight bear with acceptable risk of nonunion
- Understanding the load through the ankle joint and fixation techniques, patients can be allowed to bear weight in a short leg cast or comparable device in certain populations

DISCLOSURE

None.

REFERENCES

1. Abben KW, Sorensen MD, Waverly BJ. Immediate weightbearing after first metatarsophalangeal joint arthrodesis with screw and locking plate fixation: a short-term review. J Foot Ankle Surg 2018;57(4):771–5.
2. Prissel MA, Hyer CF, Grambart ST, et al. A multicenter, retrospective study of early weightbearing for modified lapidus arthrodesis. J Foot Ankle Surg 2016;55(2):226–9.
3. King CM, Richey J, Patel S, et al. Modified Lapidus arthrodesis with crossed screw fixation: early weightbearing in 136 patients. J Foot Ankle Surg 2015;54(1):69–75.
4. Gul A, Batra S, Mehmood S, et al. Immediate unprotected weight-bearing of operatively treated ankle fractures. Acta Orthop Belg 2007;73:360–5.
5. Dehghan N, McKee MD, Jenkinson RJ, et al. Early weight bearing and range of motion versus non-weight bearing and immobilization after open reduction and internal fixation of unstable ankle fractures: a randomized controlled trial. J Orthop Trauma 2016;30:345–52.
6. Starkweather MP, Collman DR, Schuberth JM. Early protected weight bearing after open reduction internal fixation of ankle fractures. J Foot Ankle Surg 2012;51:575–8.
7. Lynde MJ, Sautter T, Hamilton GA, et al. Complications after open reduction and internal fixation of ankle fractures in the elderly. Foot Ankle Surg 2012;18:103–7.
8. Soroceanu A, Sidhwa F, Aarabi S, et al. Surgical versus nonsurgical treatment of acute Achilles tendon rupture: a meta-analysis of randomized trials. The Journal of Bone and Joint Surgery. American volume 2012;94(23):2136.
9. Lundeen GA, Diefenbach C, Moles LH, et al. Immediate unrestricted weightbearing with simple stirrup brace following single anchor lateral ankle ligament stabilization. Foot Ankle Spec 2022;15(5):456–63.
10. Vopat ML, Wendling A, Lee B, et al. Early versus delayed mobilization postoperative protocols for primary lateral ankle ligament reconstruction: a systematic review and meta-analysis. Kansas Journal of Medicine 2021;14:141.
11. Clark BC. In vivo alterations in skeletal muscle form and function after disuse atrophy. Med Sci Sports Exerc 2009;41:1869–75.
12. Nesheiwat F, Sergi AR. Deep venous thrombosis and pulmonary embolism following cast immobilization of the lower extremity. J Foot Ankle Surg 1996;35:590–4.

13. Hyer CF, Scott RT, Swiatek M. A retrospective comparison of four plate constructs for first metatarsophalangeal joint fusion: static plate, static plate with lag screw, locked plate, and locked plate with lag screw. J Foot Ankle Surg 2012;51(3): 285–7.

14. Mayer SA, Zelenski NA, DeOrio JK, et al. A comparison of nonlocking semitubular plates and precontoured locking plates for first metatarsophalangeal joint arthrodesis. Foot Ankle Int 2014;35(5):438–44.

15. Crowell A, Van JC, Meyr AJ. Early weight-bearing after arthrodesis of the first metatarsal-phalangeal joint: a systematic review of the incidence of non-union. J Foot Ankle Surg 2018;57(6):1200–3.

16. Füssenich W, Seeber GH, Zwoferink JR, et al. Non-union incidence of different joint preparation types, joint fixation techniques, and postoperative weightbearing protocols for arthrodesis of the first metatarsophalangeal joint in moderate-to-severe hallux valgus: a systematic review. EFORT Open Rev 2023;8(3):101–9.

17. Roukis TS. Nonunion after arthrodesis of the first metatarsal-phalangeal joint: a systematic review. J Foot Ankle Surg 2011;50:710–3.

18. West TA, Pollard JD, Carpenter DM, et al. Crossed screw fixation versus dorsal plating for first metatarsophalangeal joint arthrodesis: a retrospective cohort study. J Foot Ankle Surg 2022;61(1):32–6.

19. Dayton P, Kauwe M, DiDomenico L, et al. Quantitative analysis of the degree of frontal rotation required to anatomically align the first metatarsal phalangeal joint during modified tarsal-metatarsal arthrodesis without capsular balancing. J Foot Ankle Surg 2016;55(2):220–5.

20. King CM, Hamilton GA, Ford LA. Effects of the Lapidus arthrodesis and chevron bunionectomy on plantar forefoot pressures. J Foot Ankle Surg 2014;53(4):415–9.

21. Avino A, Patel S, Hamilton GA, et al. The effect of the Lapidus arthrodesis on the medial longitudinal arch: a radiographic review. J Foot Ankle Surg 2008;47(6): 510–4.

22. Catanzariti AR, Mendicino RW, Lee MS, et al. The modified Lapidus arthrodesis: a retrospective analysis. J Foot Ankle Surg 1999;38(5):322–32.

23. Sangeorzan BJ, Hansen ST Jr. Modified Lapidus procedure for hallux valgus. Foot Ankle 1989;9(6):262–6.

24. Mcinnes BD, Bouché RT. Critical evaluation of the modified Lapidus procedure. J Foot Ankle Surg 2001;40(2):71–90.

25. Myerson M, Allon S, McGarvey W. Metatarsocuneiform arthrodesis for management of hallux valgus and metatarsus primus varus. Foot Ankle 1992;13(3): 107–15.

26. Coetzee JC, Resig SG, Kuskowski M, et al. The Lapidus procedure as salvage after failed surgical treatment of hallux valgus: a prospective cohort study. JBJS 2003;85(1):60–5.

27. Patel S, Ford LA, Etcheverry J,, et al. Modified Lapidus arthrodesis: rate of nonunion in 227 cases. J Foot Ankle Surg 2004;43(1):37–42.

28. Kraus JC, McKeon KE, Johnson JE, et al. Intraosseous and extraosseous blood supply to the medial cuneiform: implications for dorsal opening wedge plantar-flexion osteotomy. Foot Ankle Int 2014;35(4):394–400.

29. Johnson JT, Schuberth JM, Thornton SD, et al. Joint curettage arthrodesis technique in the foot: a histological analysis. J Foot Ankle Surg 2009;48(5):558–64.

30. Nester CJ, Liu AM, Ward E, et al. In vitro study of foot kinematics using a dynamic walking cadaver model. J Biomech 2007;40(9):1927–37.

31. Pirozzi K, McGuire J, Meyr AJ. Effect of variable body mass on plantar foot pressure and off-loading device efficacy. J Foot Ankle Surg 2014;53(5):588–97.

32. Cottom JM, Rigby RB. Biomechanical comparison of a locking plate with intra-plate compression screw versus locking plate with plantar interfragmentary screw for Lapidus arthrodesis: a cadaveric study. J Foot Ankle Surg 2013; 52(3):339–42.

33. Klos K, Gueorguiev B, Mückley T, et al. Stability of medial locking plate and compression screw versus two crossed screws for Lapidus arthrodesis. Foot Ankle Int 2010;31(2):158–63.

34. Klos K, Simons P, Hajduk AS, et al. Plantar versus dorsomedial locked plating for Lapidus arthrodesis: a biomechanical comparison. Foot Ankle Int 2011;32(11): 1081–5.

35. Burchard R, Massa R, Soost C, et al. Biomechanics of common fixation devices for first tarsometatarsal joint fusion—a comparative study with synthetic bones. J Orthop Surg Res 2018;13(1):1–7.

36. Ağır İ, Tunçer N, Küçükdurmaz F, et al. Functional comparison of immediate and late weight bearing after ankle bimalleolar fracture surgery. Open Orthop J 2015; 9:188–90.

37. Firoozabadi R, Harnden E, Krieg JC. Immediate weight-bearing after ankle fracture fixation. Adv Orthop 2015;2015:491976.

38. Shaffer MA, Okereke E, Esterhai JL, et al. Effects of immobilization on plantar-flexion torque, fatigue resistance, and functional ability following an ankle fracture. Phys Ther 2000;80(8):769–80.

39. Simanski CJ, Maegele M, Lefering R, et al. Functional treatment and early weight-bearing after an ankle fracture: a prospective study. J Orthop Trauma 2006;20(2): 108–14.

40. Finsen V, Saetermo R, Kibsgaard L, et al. Early postoperative weight-bearing and muscle activity in patients who have a fracture of the ankle. J Bone Joint Surg Am 1989;71A:23–7.

41. Lehtonen H, Jarvinen TL, Honkonen S, et al. Use of a cast compared with a functional ankle brace after operative treatment of an anklefracture: a prospective, randomized study. J Bone Joint Surg Am 2003;85A:205–11.

42. Ahl T, Dalen N, Holmberg S, et al. Early weight bearing of displaced ankle fractures. Acta Orthop Scand 1987;58:535–8.

43. van Laarhoven CJ, Meeuwis JD, van der Werken C. Postoperative treatment of internally fixed ankle fractures: a prospective randomised study. J Bone Joint Surg Br 1996;78B:395–9.

44. Cimino W, Ichtertz D, Slabaugh P. Early mobilization of ankle fractures after open reduction and internal fixation. Clin Orthop Relat Res 1991;267:152–6.

45. Ahl T, Dalen N, Lundberg A, et al. Early mobilization of operated on ankle fractures: prospective, controlled study of 40 bimalleolar cases. Acta Orthop Scand 1993;64:95–9.

46. Egol KA, Dolan R, Koval KJ. Functional outcome of surgery for fractures of the ankle. A prospective, randomized comparison of management in a cast or a functional brace. J Bone Joint Surg Am 2000;82:246–9.

47. Bazarov I, Peace RA, Lagaay PI, et al. Early protected weight bearing after ankle fractures in patients with diabetes mellitus. J Foot Ankle Surg 2016;56:30–3.

48. King CM, Doyle MD, Castellucci-Garza FM, et al. Early protected weightbearing after open reduction internal fixation of ankle fractures with trans-syndesmotic screws. J Foot Ankle Surg 2020;59(4):726–8.

49. Raasch WG, Larkin JJ, Draganich LF. Assessment of the posterior malleolus as a restraint to posterior subluxation of the ankle. J Bone Joint Surg Am 1992;74(8): 1201–6.

50. Fitzpatrick DC, Otto JK, McKinley TO, et al. Kinematic and contact stress analysis of posterior malleolus fractures of the ankle. J Orthop Trauma 2004;18(5):271–8.
51. Harper MC. Posterior instability of the talus: an anatomic evaluation. Foot Ankle 1989;10(1):36–9.
52. Stiehl JB, Skrade DA, Needleman RL, et al. Effect of axial load and ankle position on ankle stability. J Orthop Trauma 1993;7(1):72–7.
53. Driscoll HL, Christensen JC, Tencer AF. Contact characteristics of the ankle joint. Part 1. The normal joint. J Am Podiatr Med Assoc 1994;84(10):491–8.
54. Harper MC, Hardin G. Posterior malleolar fractures of the ankle associated with external rotation-abduction injuries. Results with and without internal fixation. J Bone Joint Surg Am 1988;70(9):1348–56.
55. Hartford JM, Gorczyca JT, McNamara JL, et al. Tibiotalar contact area. Contribution of posterior malleolus and deltoid ligament. Clin Orthop Relat Res 1995;320: 182–7.
56. Macko VW, Matthews LS, Zwirkoski P, et al. The joint-contact area of the ankle. The contribution of the posterior malleolus. J Bone Joint Surg Am 1991;73(3): 347–51.
57. Papachristou G, Efstathopoulos N, Levidiotis C, et al. Early weight bearing after posterior malleolar fractures: an experimental and prospective clinical study. J Foot Ankle Surg 2003;42(2):99–104.

Management of High-Risk Ankle Fractures

Craig E. Krcal Jr, DPM[a,b], David R. Collman, DPM[c,d,e],*

KEYWORDS

- Ankle trauma • Osteopenia • Osteoporosis • Geriatric • Elderly • Diabetes

KEY POINTS

- Ankle fractures in diabetic and elderly patients should not be managed in the same manner as their healthy counterparts.
- Careful attention to an often-unforgiving soft tissue envelope is crucial to avoid potentially catastrophic complications in these patients.
- Altered bone properties may adversely influence healing and fracture stability. Fixation constructs must be adapted accordingly.
- Transsyndesmotic screw fixation should be routinely used to stabilize ankle fractures in these patients, who frequently cannot abide by restricted weight bearing protocols.
- Early protected weight bearing in the osteopenic patient—and some diabetic patients—is safe and helps reduce injury morbidity.

BACKGROUND

Ankle fractures among the aging baby boomers and the increasing number of patients with diabetes mellitus have evolved into a colossal health care burden. The rate of such injuries is expected to escalate.[1–4] Each patient population presents unique risks for ankle fracture management. Fractures in this population can be unpredictable and deceiving. The timing of surgery, methods of osteosynthesis to facilitate primary or secondary bone healing, and time to load bearing after surgery all play a critical role for a successful patient recovery.

[a] The CORE Institute, 18444 N 25th Avenue Suite 320, Phoenix, AZ 85023, USA; [b] Kaiser San Francisco Bay Area Foot & Ankle Residency Program Alumni Class of 2023; [c] Kaiser San Francisco Bay Area Foot & Ankle Residency Program; [d] Department of Orthopedics, Podiatry, Injury, Sports Medicine; [e] Kaiser Permanente San Francisco Medical Center, 450 6th Avenue, French Campus, 5th Floor, San Francisco, CA 94118, USA
* Corresponding author. Kaiser Permanente San Francisco Medical Center, 450 6th Avenue, French Campus, 5th Floor, San Francisco, CA 94118.
E-mail address: David.Collman@kp.org

Clin Podiatr Med Surg 41 (2024) 73–101
https://doi.org/10.1016/j.cpm.2023.06.003
0891-8422/24/© 2023 Elsevier Inc. All rights reserved.

The core problem in elderly patients with fragility, osteoporotic, or age-related fractures is compromised bone. Bone in this population is characterized by diminished trabecular density and remodeling that shifts toward resorption in much of the cortices of long bones. There is no definable underlying collagen or mineral abnormality, yet there can be upwards of 50% bone loss in the fractured extremity. This manifests as soft, malleable, and/or brittle bone, frequently resulting in comminuted fractures and additional bone loss, even in low energy injuries. The physician faces limited options in fracture treatment. It can be very difficult to maintain acceptable alignment with nonoperative care. Yet satisfactory fracture stability can be difficult to achieve with standard fixation techniques.[5–7]

Diabetic patients present a similar, but oftentimes more expansive management conundrum, which can be difficult to control. These patients typically carry a host of comorbidities resulting from a hyperglycemic state, including obesity, end-stage organ damage of the peripheral nervous and cardiovascular system, as well as advanced renal disease. Hyperglycemia compromises intra- and extracellular function due to advanced glycosylation, ultimately impairing bone healing due to an imbalance of cell-to-cell communication and osteoblastic and osteoclastic instability.[8,9] Hyperglycemia decreases bone tensile strength, stiffness, and callus size. Optimizing perioperative blood glucose levels is critical to mitigate complications. Lowering HgA1c levels by just 1% has been shown to reduce surgical complication rates by 25%.[10]

Compared with patients with uncomplicated diabetes, those with complicated diabetes—uncontrolled hyperglycemia with end-stage organ dysfunction or failure—show much poorer outcomes in the surgical treatment of ankle fractures. This fragile population has an infection rate of 17% to 50%, an amputation incidence of 4% to 7%, and revision surgery is 5 times more likely.[10] In addition, traumatic events—original injury or iatrogenic insult—may produce deranged bone remodeling associated with Charcot neuroarthropathy, leading to implant failure: implant failure, subsequent deformity, wound complications, revision surgery, or amputation.[11,12]

Aside from healing potential, these 2 patient cohorts frequently present difficult social constraints as restricted weight bearing recommendations are often unreasonable. Expecting elderly individuals and/or obese diabetic patients to remain non-weight bearing is not feasible and frankly unreasonable. In the event these patients adhere to such care instructions, they may decompensate, including cardiopulmonary compromise, increasing morbidity and mortality. A number of studies have demonstrated the burden these patients, much like geriatric hip fractures, place on our health care system in ensuring safe and appropriate disposition while balancing the needs of fracture healing.[1,5,13–15] Mitigating this burden demands reconstructing the ankle joint according to sound principles in fracture mechanics and fixation, safely mobilizing the patient with close attention to healing progress, and meeting their overall rehabilitation needs.[1,3,4]

Although patients with complicated typically diabetes require a protracted period of ankle immobilization and a longer course of non-weight bearing for successful treatment, most high-risk patients with unstable ankle fractures can safely ambulate with proper ankle protection following open reduction internal fixation (ORIF). Allowance for early protected load is rooted in ankle fracture pathomechanics. Most ankle fractures result from low-energy rotational injuries due to excessive external rotation under axial load, producing a distal fibular fracture, often with neighboring fractures or ligament disruption. Following restoration of the ankle mortise, a short leg cast or CAM boot orthosis is effective to offload the malleoli by restraining morbid rotation

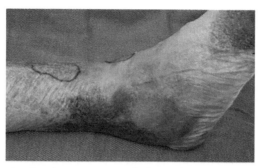

Fig. 1. Elderly patients often have tenuous soft tissues, increasing the risk for wound complications in unstable ankle fractures.

of the talus within the mortise. The cast or boot establishes vertical load, transferring force from the foot directly through the talus and plafond, thereby protecting reduction and fixation of the malleoli.[16] There is ample literature to support safe early weight bearing and range of motion following surgical treatment of unstable ankle fractures.[16–20]

Careful attention to the soft tissue envelope is paramount for the surgical treatment of ankle fractures in these patient populations. In the elderly patient, the skin is often very thin, easily bruised, and prone to tearing (**Fig 1**). Significant atrophy of the subcutaneous tissue is common. The fragile soft tissue envelope demands close attention relative to timing of surgery, tissue handling, and postoperative care.[5–7] Peripheral vascular disease and neuropathy may be present in some elderly patients, disorders that may have a devastating impact on soft tissue healing. Ankle fractures in patients with diabetes often present with both peripheral arterial disease and neuropathy. The astute surgeon takes a careful history and physical examination. Atrophic skin changes may be seen in the diabetic patient, but the more common concern is incision healing complications due to glycosylation and peripheral arterial disease.

Principles of ankle ORIF of these 2 high-risk patient populations are identical to the tenants of the Association for the Study of Internal Fixation (ASIF) in patients of lower risk: restore a congruent and stable ankle joint mortise with as little insult to soft tissue as possible and provide for early and safe mobilization. However, fixation methods to achieve these endpoints can be different. Over the last several decades there have been many advancements in ankle fracture fixation techniques, implant development, and changing perspectives on joint sparing and destructive procedures. Conventional fixation applied in a rationale and mechanically sound fashion has shown to produce equal—and at times superior—results to newer devices or techniques, even in the osteoporotic ankle.[7,19–22] These techniques rely on biomechanical principles of implant application to maximize stability. The operative techniques and treatment philosophy presented highlight methods to achieve reliable outcomes in these patient populations.

OSTEOPENIC AND ELDERLY ANKLE FRACTURE FIXATION TECHNIQUES
Tissue handling and bone healing concepts

Ankle soft tissues are often at high risk for wounds owing to fracture instability and skin tenting. It is imperative to reduce unstable ankle fractures immediately and apply a well-molded splint without excessive padding, which helps maintain the reduction. This will help minimize soft tissue compromise and avoid long delays prior to surgery. Maintaining satisfactory ankle fracture alignment in a splint over time can be difficult. During the operation, creation of multiple soft tissue planes, undermining, or significant tension on the skin should be avoided. Full thickness flaps should be raised with atraumatic soft tissue handling through an incision of appropriate length. Skin edge necrosis may be unavoidable in some instances (**Fig 2**). Close monitoring of these patients in the acute postoperative period should be considered.

Bone stability and blood supply—the 2 elements essential for bone healing—should be carefully considered during ankle ORIF in this population. Callus formation in secondary bone healing may be desirable, particularly in comminuted fractures that demand respect for the injury zone and periosteal blood supply. It is critical to avoid soft tissue stripping in the zone of injury when approaching these fractures. Stability is often adequate with bridge plating methods. The risk of devascularization with substantial dissection is often not worth primary fracture healing and should be avoided.

Poor soft tissues in the very elderly may preclude open approaches to fracture repair (**Figs. 3** and **4**). Closed reduction with percutaneous pinning may be sufficient

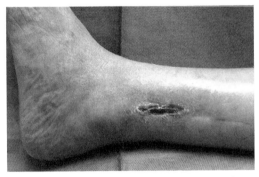

Fig. 2. Incision skin margin necrosis may occur in elderly patients after ankle fracture repair.

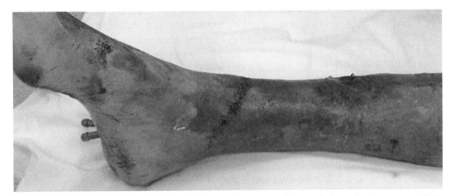

Fig. 3. Open approaches to ankle fracture repair may not be possible owing to poor soft tissues in some elderly patients. (*Courtesy of* Brian Elliot, DPM.)

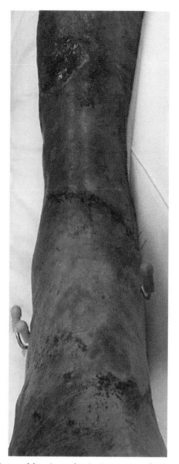

Fig. 4. Same patient, anterior ankle view depicting open fracture laceration repair.

for stability in some cases. This 85 year old woman with a history of peripheral arterial disease and atrial fibrillation with long-standing coumadin anticoagulation sustained an open bimalleolar ankle fracture dislocation. Following fracture reduction and early intravenous antibiotics, the wounds were irrigated and primarily closed. Percutaneous fixation was accomplished with an array of Steinman pins spanning the fractures (see **Figs. 3** and **4**; **Fig. 5**). Large transarticular pins were driven across the tibiotalar joint to help maintain stability during fracture healing. When using this technique, the pins should be introduced into the posterior tibiotalar joint to minimize articular insult and to engage the tibial cortex in the denser, diaphyseal bone (see **Fig 5**). The talus may also be plantarflexed to minimize damage to its articular surface.

Figs. 6 and **7** depict both primary and secondary bone healing of the fibula in an osteopenic comminuted ankle fracture suffered by a 44 year old woman with B-cell lymphoma and a contralateral nonoperative ankle fracture. An interfragmentary screw was placed across the primary fibular fracture without periosteal stripping and the larger zone of comminution was not opened, with supraperiosteal plating

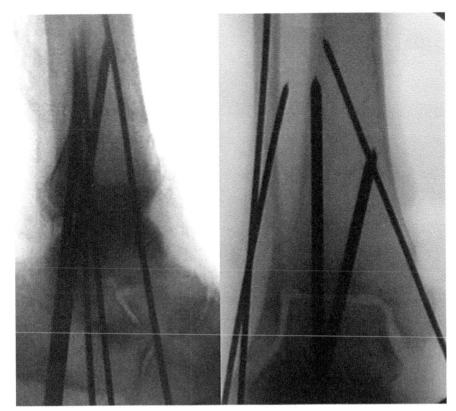

Fig. 5. Fluoroscopic images depicting transarticular pin stabilization. Note pins cross posterior tibiotalar joint to minimize articular insult.

to help preserve blood supply. A syndesmosis screw was placed to lend further support to the fibula (see below). This patient was casted on the operating room table, walked on her ankle immediately, and recovered relatively quickly. Intact mortise and fibula fracture callus formation is seen in the 2 month follow-up films (see **Fig 7**).

Antiglide plating

Antiglide plating in osteoporotic ankle fractures has its primary application in the spiral oblique distal fibular fracture and tibial fractures that tend to fail under axial loading with shearing forces. There are clear mechanical advantages to antiglide plating with conventional implants for fixation of distal fibular fractures compared with neutralization plating and locking plates.[23–26] Posterolateral plating of the distal fibula is the workhorse of osteopenic fractures, effectively preventing superior, posterior, and lateral migration of the distal fibula fragment. Soft tissue coverage is also superior compared with lateral plating methods. This technique produces good results in soft bone.[23–27]

Fig. 8 depicts a 70 year old man with a trimalleolar ankle fracture equivalent (deltoid lesion). Following posterolateral plating of the fibula, the talus was effectively incarcerated in the mortise. In some instances, diaphyseal bone strength is sufficient

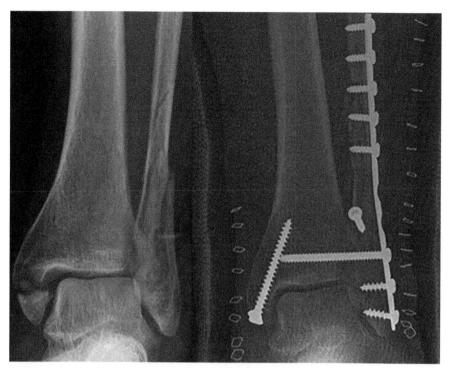

Fig. 6. Osteopenic bimalleolar ankle fracture. The comminuted fibular fracture zone was spanned to avoid compromising periosteal blood supply. Syndesmosis screw helps support fibula.

to maintain construct stability. This patient required only minimum screw fixation because his bone was relatively strong. This patient was managed non-weight bearing in a splint for 10 days, transitioned to a walking cast for 3.5 weeks, followed by a fracture boot for 2 weeks, before progressing into regular shoes roughly 6 weeks after surgery as radiographs demonstrated fracture healing and an intact mortise (**Fig. 9**).

Posterolateral plating of the distal fibula also permits bicortical purchase of all screws that secure the plate to bone, increasing construct stability compared with unicortical distal metaphyseal screw placement in lateral plating methods. The metaphysis can be drilled with a 2.0 mm Steinman pin to improve screw thread purchase. **Fig. 10** depicts bicortical purchase of the distal metaphyseal bone of the fibula in an 82 year old woman. This screw frequently measures between 24 and 28 mm in length as the distal fibula widens. Finally, the technique does not preclude placement of transsyndesmotic fixation, as shown below.

Antiglide plating is also useful for larger posterior malleolar fractures often seen in low-energy injuries in this population. **Fig. 11** depicts a 74 year old woman with controlled diabetes who sustained a comminuted trimalleolar ankle fracture with a posteromedial malleolar fracture involving roughly 25% of the plafond (see **Fig 11**). Antiglide plates were applied to both the fibula and the tibia with the addition of a syndesmosis screw, stabilizing the talus against posterior escape (**Fig. 12**). Small screws were used to stabilize the small comminuted medial malleolar fracture. This patient

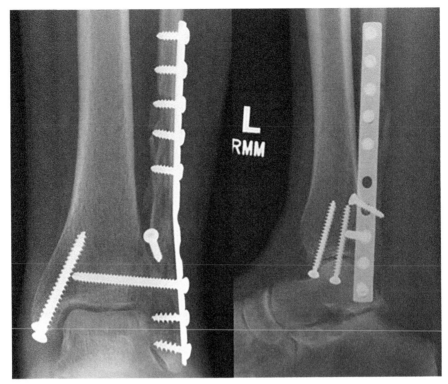

Fig. 7. Postoperative radiographs of the same patient 2 months later. The patient walked in a short leg cast immediately after surgery. The mortise remained intact. Note fibula callus formation.

was permitted to walk in a short leg cast within 10 days of surgery and went on to uneventful healing. In some cases, screw fixation is adequate to stabilize larger posterior malleolar fractures in the elderly population and should be placed close to the joint to capture more bone (see **Fig 10**). Early load is permitted in most posterior malleolar fractures because neutral ankle alignment afforded by the cast or boot puts the talar contact pressure at the center of the plafond, so the posterior malleolar fragment does not load.[28]

Syndesmotic fixation/fibula pro-tibia screw stabilization

Placement of syndesmosis screws in this population is common because it enhances construct stability, regardless of syndesmosis injury. In cases of appreciable osteopenia and fracture comminution, multiple syndesmotic screws should be placed through a plate and purchase 4 cortices. When combined with a stiff plate, or stacked traditional plates, this technique significantly increases the stiffness of the construct as the fibula buttresses the talus under the tibia.[28,29] This technique provides excellent control of the fibular segment.

Fig. 13 depicts a 74 year old man with cardiac disease, idiopathic neuropathy, and osteopenia who presented with a highly comminuted distal fibular fracture and deltoid ligament compromise. Stability was attained with interfragmentary screws of the

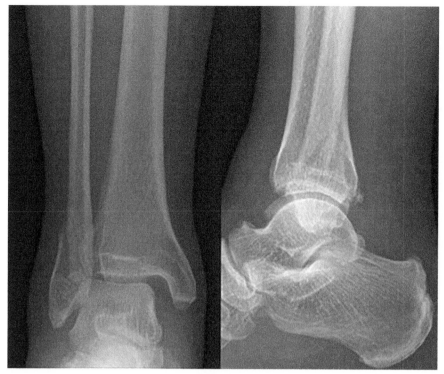

Fig. 8. Trimalleolar ankle fracture equivalent (deltoid lesion) in an elderly man.

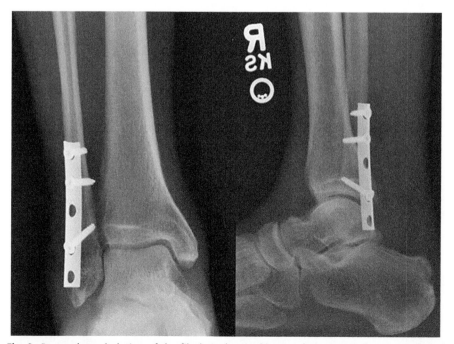

Fig. 9. Posterolateral plating of the fibula is the workhorse of osteopenic fractures. Healed fracture and intact mortise 6 weeks after surgery, early weight bearing in short cast.

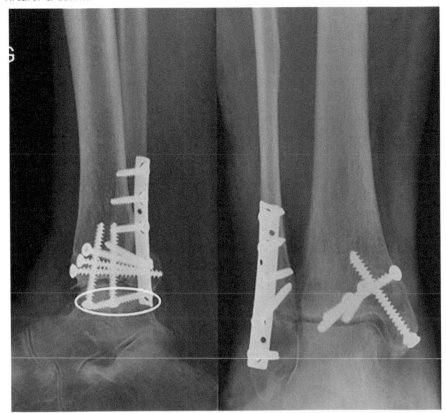

Fig. 10. Posterolateral plating of the fibula allows for distal bicortical screw purchase, producing a more stable fixation construct in osteopenic fractures.

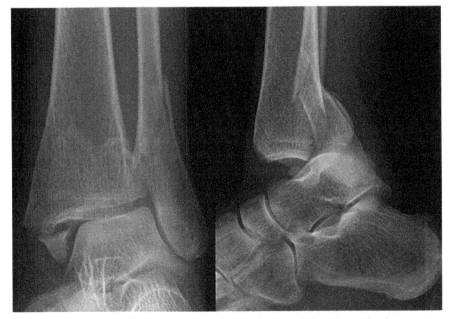

Fig. 11. Osteopenic trimalleolar comminuted ankle fracture dislocation with a large posteromedial fragment in an elderly woman.

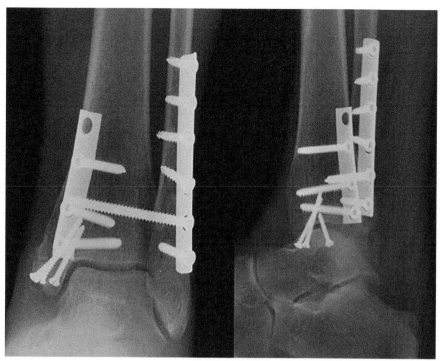

Fig. 12. Postoperative radiographs in the same patient, stabilized with antiglide plating of the tibia/fibula and a syndesmosis screw to prevent posterior escape of the talus.

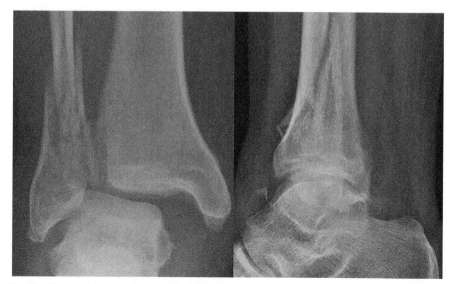

Fig. 13. Osteopenic comminuted distal fibular ankle fracture with deltoid compromise in an elderly man with neuropathy.

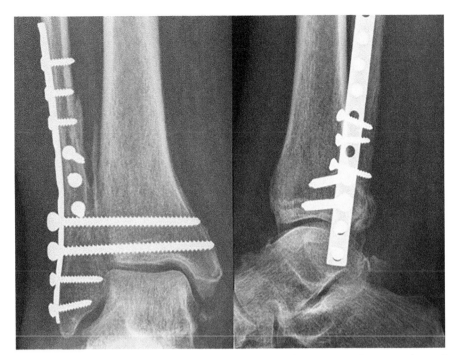

Fig. 14. Ankle radiographs at 5 months in the same patient. Large 4.5 mm syndesmosis screws significantly increase construct stiffness and are routinely used in this patient population, even when the syndesmosis is not compromised.

primary fracture, conventional neutralization plating, and stout 4.5 mm quadracortical syndesmotic screws. Radiographs at 5 months demonstrate a healed fibula and talus maintained in the mortise (**Fig 14**). This technique is routinely used in our institutions for both osteopenic and neuropathic ankle fractures alike, particularly when postoperative recommendations for non-weight bearing are assumed to be unmet in the latter population.

Intramedullary pins

This technique is well documented in the literature and is particularly useful in severe osteopenic ankle fractures where screws will purchase. Osteopenic bone has a predictably lower volume of trabecular bone with weakened cortices. Intramedullary pins add to the intracortical mass, incarcerating the fibular fragment (**Fig. 15**). The screw-pin interference augments bending and torsional stability.[28–30] The pins should be driven past the fracture, well into the diaphysis, and are typically placed after fracture reduction. A plate is then secured with screws to complete the construct. In some cases, passing the drill and screws along the pins may engage them, advancing the pins up the fibular diaphysis. This problem can be avoided by bending the end of the pins or clamping them at the entrance of the fibula. Alternatively, the pins can be driven after plate/screw application, though this can be more technically challenging. Such constructs permit early load in a short leg cast or boot.

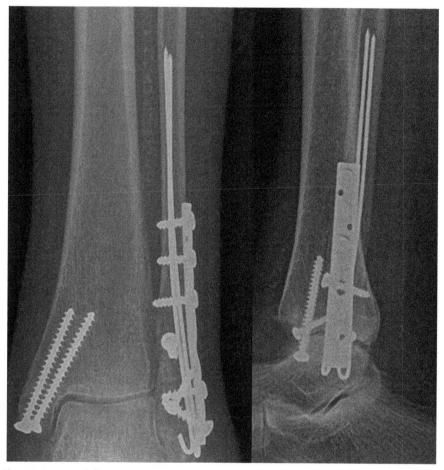

Fig. 15. Intramedullary pins improve construct stability in bending and torsion for osteopenic fibular fractures.

Tension band wiring

Tension band wiring has a storied history in fracture management. It is particularly useful in short, transverse fractures of the distal fibula and the medial malleolus, especially small collicular fragments. The added benefits of this technique in the osteoporotic fracture include adjustable tensioning, multiple points of fixation through multiple cortices, and direct buttressing of any focal comminution at the major fracture line. A transverse 3.5 mm bicortical hang screw for the wire is stronger than a bone tunnel in the osteopenic fracture (**Fig. 16**).[31] A bone tunnel risks failure in soft bone if the wire is overtightened.

Hook plate

Manufactured plates designed for a single function tend to be expensive, nonconforming, and can be oversized on the medial malleolus. They are stiff and resist tension failure but are often too bulky to use in fragile skin envelopes. When called for, a

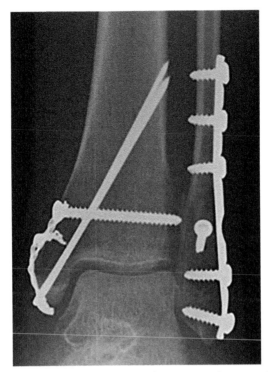

Fig. 16. Tension band wiring with transverse hang screw is a good choice for small bone fragments in the osteopenic ankle fracture. The screw is stronger than a bone tunnel for wire tightening. The pins should be driven into far cortex for optimal stability.

standard 1/3 semi-tubular plate may be fashioned into a hook plate with a robust wire cutter and bent into shape with pilers. The sharp end of the plate is tamped into the distal fibula or medial malleolus with the option to add an axial screw, as depicted in **Fig. 17**.

DIABETIC ANKLE FRACTURE FIXATION TECHNIQUES

Many of the techniques described for osteopenic ankle fractures are also used in diabetic ankle fractures because they achieve the most stable constructs for the respective fracture patterns. Aside from deranged bone turnover and the untoward effects of hyperglycemia in the diabetic patient population, special attention must be given to inevitable challenges with non-weight bearing in cases of obesity and neuropathy.

Super constructs in foot and ankle surgery are often associated with Charcot reconstruction but are also well suited to many diabetic ankle fractures. In 1995, Schon recommended multiple tetracortical syndesmosis screws along with a prolonged period of ankle immobilization and non-weight bearing.[32] Wukich and colleagues[33] evaluated more robust fixation methods for ankle fractures in complicated diabetic patients and found that "ORIF Plus" techniques with multiple large trans-syndesmotic screws—and in some cases, large transarticular Steinman

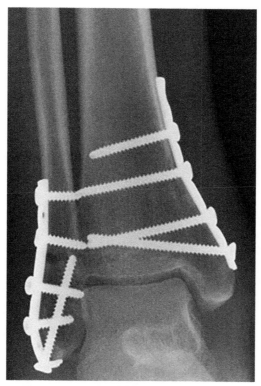

Fig. 17. Custom semi-tubular hook plates conform to bone well and are often a better choice over manufactured hook plates in the elderly patient with a tension-failure fibula fracture and thin skin envelope.

pins—resulted in fewer complications. Although the fracture patterns seen in this patient population are often no different than those seen in their nondiabetic counterparts, catastrophic failure may result when simple methods of additional fixation to establish a robust construct are ignored. The absence of syndesmosis screws can quickly produce early failure in this high-risk population, even in uncomplicated fracture patterns (**Figs. 18** and **19**). Standard 1/3 semi-tubular plating with numerous 4.5 mm quadracortical transsyndesmotic screws and a longer period of ankle immobilization are often adequate to maintain ankle stability in diabetic patients who are morbidly obese, neuropathic, or ignore postoperative non-weight bearing restrictions. Dynamic compression plates may also be used instead of of semi-tubular plates.

Fig. 20 demonstrates the super construct principle in a typical Weber B bimalleolar equivalent fracture. This patient was a 57 year old severely obese male with congestive heart failure and long-standing type 2 diabetes with peripheral neuropathy. He was treated with a multiple 4.5 mm syndesmotic screw "ladder" through a 1/3 semi-tubular plate with maintenance of the mortise at 9 month follow-up. Note the heterotopic ossification at the medial/distal tibial metaphysis and throughout the syndesmosis, highlighting the alteration of bone remodeling in these patients.

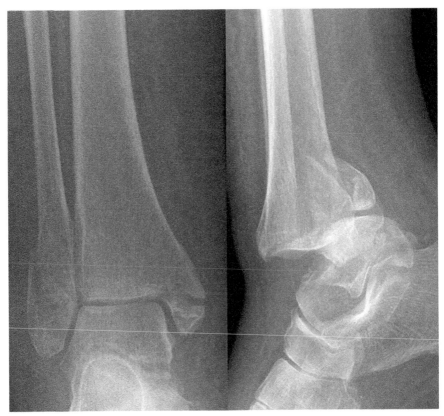

Fig. 18. Trimalleolar ankle fracture in severely obese patient with insulin-dependent poorly controlled diabetes and dense neuropathy.

Figs. 21–23 depict the same principle and illustrate the importance of prompt closed reduction and splinting to minimize soft tissue insult in this population. This densely neuropathic, severely obese 64 year old man with alcoholic cirrhosis and controlled type 2 diabetes sustained a trimalleolar ankle fracture equivalent (see **Fig. 21**). It took a week for his soft tissues to quiesce in skilled care as a robust well-molded splint maintained the reduction (see **Fig. 22**). ORIF was achieved with a 4.5 mm screw syndesmotic ladder through a 1/3 semi-tubular plate. He was asked to remain non-weight bearing in a short leg cast thereafter. Six weeks after surgery his cast showed signs of wear, but the ankle mortise was intact (see **Fig. 23**). Six months later, he was deceased.

Fig. 24 depicts a comminuted trimalleolar fracture dislocation in a 64 year old severely obese man with congestive heart failure, neuropathy, and poorly controlled diabetes (HgA1c 9%). The posterior malleolar fracture was reduced with the fibula but not fixed because the syndesmosis screws provided adequate stability. The zone of injury in the fibula was not disrupted during the approach and spanned with stacked 1/3 semi-tubular plates to increase construct rigidity (**Fig. 25**). This patient managed to stay off his ankle in a cast for 2.5 months as advised. The patient required a year for full recovery and did well.

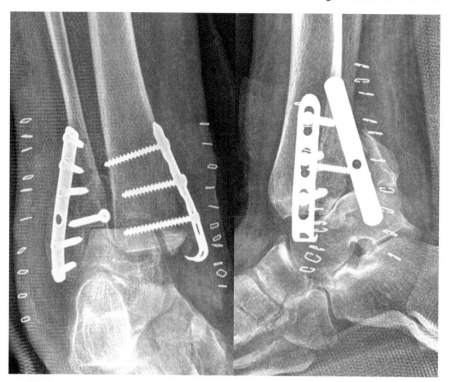

Fig. 19. Postoperative radiographs of same patient depict early failure within 2 weeks of surgery at another medical center. Note the absence of syndesmosis screws, which may have prevented re-dislocation. The patient developed a large anterior distal tibial wound and eventually required below-knee amputation.

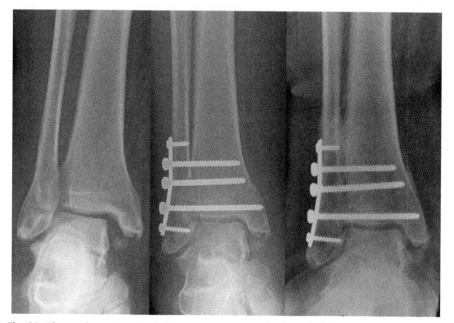

Fig. 20. The syndesmosis screw ladder superconstruct effectively stabilizes common ankle fracture patterns and produces favorable outcomes in patients with diabetic peripheral neuropathy.

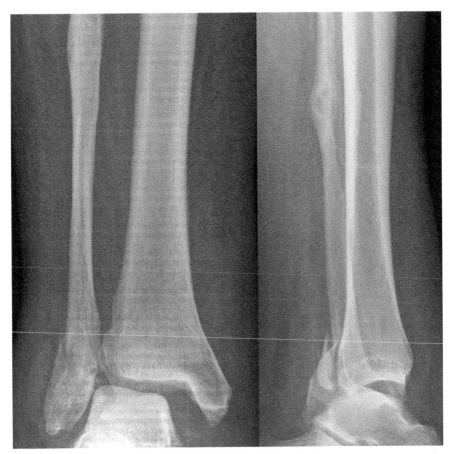

Fig. 21. Trimalleolar ankle fracture in a severely obese diabetic man with dense neuropathy.

Closed reduction and percutaneous delivery of implants may be indicated for unstable ankle fractures in very high-risk patients who have numerous comorbidities and need to ambulate early to avoid cardiopulmonary decompensation. **Figs. 26–28** illustrate this approach in an elderly patient with poorly controlled diabetes, end-stage renal disease on hemodialysis, extensive cardiac disease, chronic respiratory failure, and prior ipsilateral toe amputation. Little more than stab incisions were necessary to insert the plate and screws. The patient walked in a short leg cast within 2 weeks of surgery.

Charcot neuroarthropathy can produce significant morbidity in the ankle. A 77 year old female with early dementia and long-standing type 2 diabetes presented with a red, warm, and swollen ankle that was grossly unstable (**Fig. 29**). Elements of her history were unclear, but she may have had pedal osteomyelitis a few years prior. She had palpable pedal pulses and dense neuropathy to the leg. Work-up for infection was unremarkable and she was placed in a short leg cast for 6 weeks with close monitoring until the acute Charcot event subsided. She underwent primary tibiotalar arthrodesis with morselized fibular autogenous graft, stabilized with ring fixator over 3 months (**Fig. 30**). The fusion mass was stable when the fixator was removed,

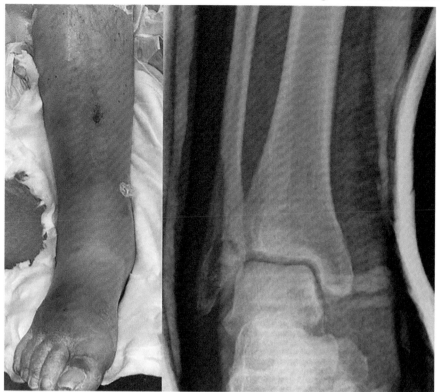

Fig. 22. Significant soft tissue inflammation in the same patient. Fracture reduction was maintained in a robust, well-molded splint.

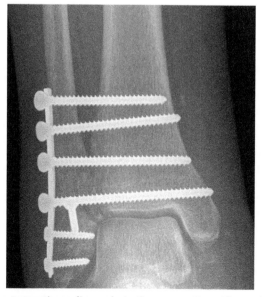

Fig. 23. Six-week postoperative radiographs in the same patient. The syndesmosis screw ladder helped to maintain an intact mortise despite the patient walking in the cast.

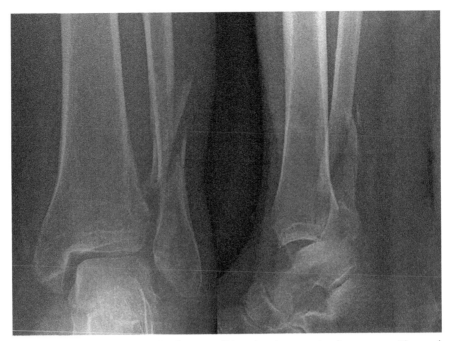

Fig. 24. Comminuted trimalleolar fracture dislocation in severely obese man with poorly controlled diabetes and peripheral neuropathy.

demonstrated on stress fluoroscopy (**Fig. 31**). Her 9-month postoperative films showed a solid fusion mass (**Fig. 32**). She walked without a brace, requiring only a cane.

OUTCOMES AND DISCUSSION

The core principles of ankle fracture management in both osteopenic and diabetic patients are initial soft tissue and medical management, early time to ORIF with adequate fixation, and protected weight bearing as soon as it is reasonable to prevent decompensation and morbidity.

The safe surgical treatment of elderly patients with unstable ankle fractures has been established.[34] Although prolonged immobilization in this population is recommended, the safety of early protected weight bearing has not been widely evaluated. One study from our institution over a decade ago retrospectively evaluated 216 patients over the age of 60 years with surgical ankle fractures requiring ORIF, with at least 6 months of follow-up.[19] Of these patients, 45 underwent ORIF with conventional plating methods and were allowed to weight bear with cast protection within 2 weeks; only a single patient experienced hardware failure. Overall complication rates peaked at 18.18% in patients with co-morbidities compared with 10.87% in those without. The most common complication was wound dehiscence.

More recently, techniques of both fibular intramedullary nailing and tibiotalocalcaneal (TTC) nailing with early weight bearing in elderly ankle fractures have been introduced.[35,36] Fibular nailing should be reserved for cases of significant soft tissue

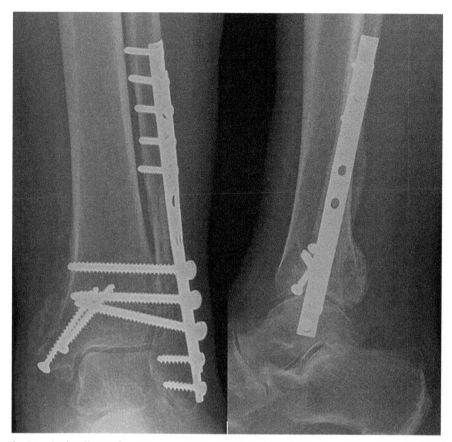

Fig. 25. Final radiographs at 1 year in the same patient illustrating the techniques of stacked fibular plating for improved stability, a syndesmosis screw ladder, and spanning the zone of fibular fracture comminution.

impairment. We have not found TTC nailing necessary because of good outcomes with joint-preservation surgery. In fact, a recent randomized controlled trial demonstrated a higher complication rate and need for second surgery in TTC nailing compared with standard ORIF techniques.[37] However, TTC nailing may be necessary for limb salvage in some complex diabetic ankle fractures or those complicated by Charcot.[38,39]

The successful treatment of operative diabetic ankle fractures requires adherence to established principles of internal fixation and prolonged immobilization. A systematic review evaluated the outcomes of standard ankle fracture fixation in diabetic patients versus alternative fixation modalities—percutaneous and minimally invasive techniques (MIS)—in 11 studies.[15] There were 420 total diabetic ankle fractures: 326 standard ORIF, 80 percutaneous/MIS, and 14 combined. The predicted odds of hardware failure or migration in MIS techniques were compared with standard fixation, concluding that improved salvage rates correlate with the practice of standard internal fixation principles along with judicious glycemic control and prolonged immobilization. Literature in our institution demonstrates similar findings but

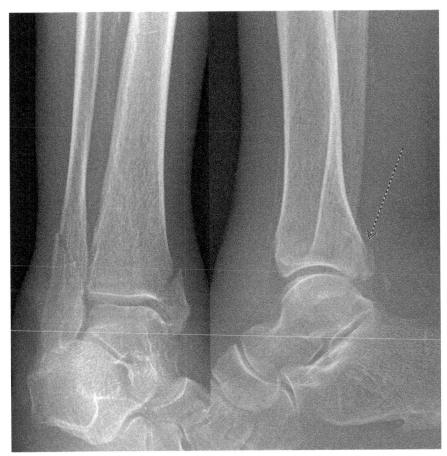

Fig. 26. Minimally displaced trimalleolar ankle fracture in very high-risk elderly patient with complicated diabetes and peripheral arterial disease.

advocates for early protected weight bearing in select diabetic patients with fewer comorbidities: 73 patients with diabetes underwent ORIF of their ankle fracture with standard internal fixation methods and were kept non-weight bearing for an average of 2 weeks, followed by weight bearing in a short leg cast or boot for 4 to 6 weeks. The most common complication was wound dehiscence or surgical site infection, but only 4.2% of patients had deep infections and no patient experienced limb amputation or death within 6 months of surgery.[40] However, in patients with complicated diabetes or those with dense neuropathy, an initial period of non-weight bearing in cast or brace and an extensive period of protected weight bearing may be necessary.[10,32]

Lastly, the medical management of osteopenia in the elderly patient cannot be overlooked. Bone health must be carefully evaluated in each patient: query for prior fragility fracture, reference existing bone mineral density scan, and inquire about medications for osteoporosis.[41] Laboratory studies should include 25-hydroxyvitamin D, serum calcium, alkaline phosphatase, parathyroid hormone,

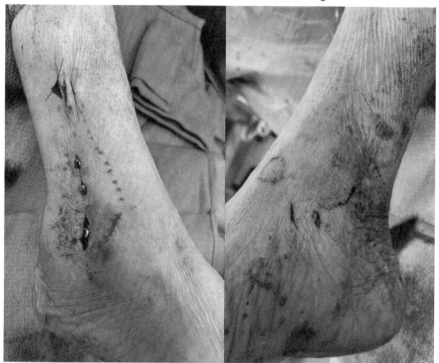

Fig. 27. Intraoperative photographs demonstrate the minimally invasive fracture approach in the same patient. A key elevator established a subcutaneous tunnel for the fibular plate.

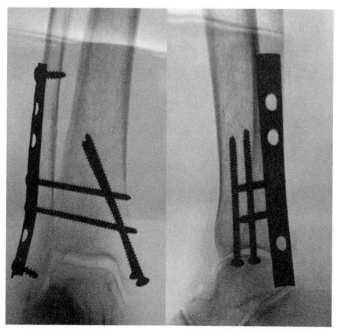

Fig. 28. Postoperative radiographs of the same patient depict minimal plate and screw osteosynthesis for sufficient fracture stability. The patient was permitted to walk in a short leg cast within 2 weeks of surgery and did well. (Courtesy of Lawrence Ford, DPM.)

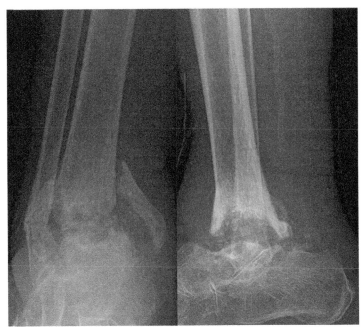

Fig. 29. Acute ankle Charcot neuroarthropathy with marked collapse and bone resorption of the tibial plafond/talar body in this elderly woman.

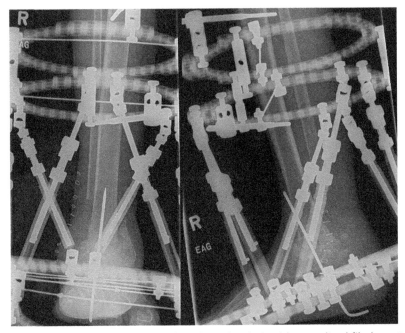

Fig. 30. The same patient underwent tibiotalar arthrodesis with morselized fibular autogenous graft and ring fixator stabilization once the acute Charcot event subsided. (In collaboration with Jack Schuberth, DPM.)

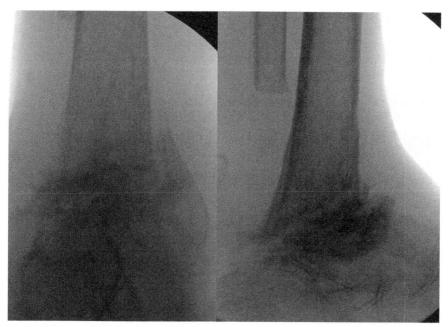

Fig. 31. Fluoroscopic stress imaging demonstrates stable fusion mass after fixator removal in the same patient.

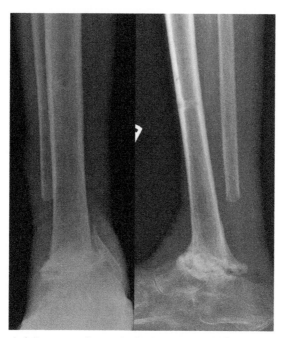

Fig. 32. Nine month follow-up radiographs in the same patient. The fusion mass was solid and she was able to walk without a brace, cane-assisted.

and thyroid-stimulating hormone. Fall prevention and strengthening programs, reducing alcohol use, and stopping medications that may be responsible for bone loss are important. High-quality randomized controlled trials have demonstrated the efficacy of bisphosphonates for fracture prevention in osteoporotic patients.[42–44] The primary care physician and endocrinologist should collaborate on optimizing bone health to minimize the risk of additional fragility fractures. Finally, although vitamin D supplementation is often recommended in this population, our understanding about the efficacy of this treatment in fragility fracture management and prevention remains incomplete. A recent high-quality large randomized controlled trial demonstrated no significant effect in nonvertebral fractures in patients randomized to vitamin D supplementation compared with placebo counterparts.[45]

SUMMARY

Deficiencies in bone strength, fracture healing, soft tissue resilience, and host comorbidities in elderly and diabetic patients create significant challenges for the treatment of unstable ankle fractures. Patients in these high-risk groups should not be managed in the same manner as their healthy counterparts. Our experience with the treatment of these patients demonstrates satisfactory and predictable outcomes with the rational application of internal fixation principles and early cast or brace protected weight bearing in select patient groups.

CLINICS CARE POINTS

- Osteopenic and diabetic ankle fractures often present complex treatment challenges because of tenuous soft tissue, bone derangement, and host compromise.
- Prompt ankle fracture reduction and splint or cast stabilization, with careful attention to the soft tissue envelope, is the essential first step in treatment.
- Internal fixation constructs should be based on fracture mechanics and bone strength. Super constructs—most often transsyndemotic screws—are often necessary for adequate stability and prevention of failure in patients with ankle fractures.
- Expect complications, particularly in patients with complicated diabetes.
- Early protected weight bearing after ankle fracture repair is advisable for all patients except those with dense neuropathy or complicated diabetes.

DISCLOSURE

None.

REFERENCES

1. Kadakia RJ, Hsu RY, Hayda R, et al. Evaluation of one-year mortality after geriatric ankle fractures in patients admitted to nursing homes. Injury 2015;46(10): 2010–5.
2. Gauthé R, Desseaux A, Rony L, et al. Ankle fractures in the elderly: treatment and results in 477 patients. Orthop Traumatol Surg Res 2016;102(4 Suppl):S241–4.
3. Kadakia RJ, Ahearn BM, Tenenbaum S, et al. Costs associated with geriatric ankle fractures. Foot Ankle Spec 2017;10(1):26–30.

4. Spek RWA, Smeeing DPJ, van den Heuvel L, et al. Complications after surgical treatment of geriatric ankle fractures. J Foot Ankle Surg 2021;60(4):712–7.

5. Hollensteiner M, Sandriesser S, Bliven E, et al. Biomechanics of osteoporotic fracture fixation. Curr Osteoporos Rep 2019;17(6):363–74.

6. Pearce O, Al-Hourani K, Kelly M. Ankle fractures in the elderly: current concepts. Injury 2020;51(12):2740–7.

7. Hsu RY, Ramirez JM, Blankenhorn BD. Surgical considerations for osteoporosis in ankle fracture fixation. Orthop Clin North Am 2019;50(2):245–58.

8. Murray CE, Coleman CM. Impact of diabetes mellitus on bone health. Int J Mol Sci 2019;20(19):4873.

9. Polachek WS, Baker HP, Dahm JS, et al. Diabetic kidney disease is associated with increased complications following operative management of ankle fractures. Foot Ankle Orthop 2022;7(3). 24730114221112106.

10. Wukich DK, Kline AJ. The management of ankle fractures in patients with diabetes. J Bone Joint Surg Am 2008;90(7):1570–8.

11. Lavery LA, Lavery DC, Green T, et al. Increased risk of nonunion and Charcot arthropathy after ankle fracture in people with diabetes. J Foot Ankle Surg 2020;59(4):653–6.

12. Gougoulias N, Oshba H, Dimitroulias A, et al. Ankle fractures in diabetic patients. EFORT Open Rev 2020;5(8):457–63.

13. Toole WP, Elliott M, Hankins D, et al. Are low-energy open ankle fractures in the elderly the new geriatric hip fracture? J Foot Ankle Surg 2015;54(2):203–6.

14. Manway JM, Blazek CD, Burns PR. Special considerations in the management of diabetic ankle fractures. Curr Rev Musculoskelet Med 2018;11(3):445–55.

15. Manchanda K, Nakonezny P, Sathy AK, et al. A systematic review of ankle fracture treatment modalities in diabetic patients [published correction appears in J Clin Orthop Trauma. 2021 Aug 05;21:101558]. J Clin Orthop Trauma 2020; 16:7–15.

16. Tan EW, Sirisreetreerux N, Paez AG, et al. Early weightbearing after operatively treated ankle fractures: a biomechanical analysis. Foot Ankle Int 2016;37(6): 652–8.

17. Dehghan N, McKee MD, Jenkinson RJ, et al. Early weightbearing and range of motion versus non-weightbearing and immobilization after open reduction and internal fixation of unstable ankle fractures: a randomized controlled trial. J Orthop Trauma 2016;30(7):345–52. https://doi.org/10.1097/BOT.0000000000000572.

18. King CM, Doyle MD, Castellucci-Garza FM, et al. Early protected weightbearing after open reduction internal fixation of ankle fractures with trans-syndesmotic screws. J Foot Ankle Surg 2020;59(4):726–8. https://doi.org/10.1053/j.jfas.2020. 01.003.

19. Lynde MJ, Sautter T, Hamilton GA, et al. Complications after open reduction and internal fixation of ankle fractures in the elderly. Foot Ankle Surg 2012;18(2): 103–7. https://doi.org/10.1016/j.fas.2011.03.010.

20. Starkweather MP, Collman DR, Schuberth JM. Early protected weightbearing after open reduction internal fixation of ankle fractures. J Foot Ankle Surg 2012; 51(5):575–8.

21. Davis AT, Israel H, Cannada LK, et al. A biomechanical comparison of one-third tubular plates versus periarticular plates for fixation of osteoporotic distal fibula fractures. J Orthop Trauma 2013;27(9):e201–7.

22. Deng Y, Staniforth TL, Zafar MS, et al. Posterior antiglide plating vs lateral neutralization plating for weber b distal fibular fractures: a systematic review and meta-analysis of clinical and biomechanical studies. Foot Ankle Int 2022;43(6):850–9.

23. Schaffer JJ, Manoli A 2nd. The antiglide plate for distal fibular fixation. A biomechanical comparison with fixation with a lateral plate. J Bone Joint Surg Am 1987; 69(4):596–604.
24. Winkler B, Weber BG, Simpson LA. The dorsal antiglide plate in the treatment of Danis-Weber type-B fractures of the distal fibula. Clin Orthop Relat Res 1990;259: 204–9.
25. Minihane KP, Lee C, Ahn C, et al. Comparison of lateral locking plate and antiglide plate for fixation of distal fibular fractures in osteoporotic bone: a biomechanical study. J Orthop Trauma 2006;20(8):562–6.
26. Nguyentat A, Camisa W, Patel S, et al. A biomechanical comparison of locking versus conventional plate fixation for distal fibula fractures in trimalleolar ankle injuries. J Foot Ankle Surg 2016;55(1):132–5.
27. Driscoll HL, Christensen JC, Tencer AF. Contact characteristics of the ankle joint. Part 1. The normal joint. J Am Podiatr Med Assoc 1994;84(10):491–8.
28. Bevan WP, Barei DP, Nork SE. Operative fixation of osteoporotic ankle fractures. Tech Foot Ankle Surg 2006;5(4):222–9.
29. Koval KJ, Petraco DM, Kummer FJ, et al. A new technique for complex fibula fracture fixation in the elderly: a clinical and biomechanical evaluation. J Orthop Trauma 1997;11(1):28–33.
30. Dunn WR, Easley ME, Parks BG, et al. An augmented fixation method for distal fibular fractures in elderly patients: a biomechanical evaluation. Foot Ankle Int 2004;25(3):128–31.
31. Georgiadis GM, White DB. Modified tension band wiring of medial malleolar ankle fractures. Foot Ankle Int 1995;16(2):64–8.
32. Schon LC, Marks RM. The management of neuroarthropathic fracture-dislocations in the diabetic patient. Orthop Clin North Am 1995;26(2):375–92.
33. Wukich DK, Joseph A, Ryan M, et al. Outcomes of ankle fractures in patients with uncomplicated versus complicated diabetes. Foot Ankle Int 2011;32(2):120–30.
34. Koval KJ, Zhou W, Sparks MJ, et al. Complications after ankle fracture in elderly patients. Foot Ankle Int 2007;28(12):1249–55.
35. Coifman O, Bariteau JT, Shazar N, et al. Lateral malleolus closed reduction and internal fixation with intramedullary fibular rod using minimal invasive approach for the treatment of ankle fractures. Foot Ankle Surg 2019;25(1):79–83.
36. Large TM, Kaufman AM, Frisch HM, et al. High-risk ankle fractures in high-risk older patients: to fix or nail? [published online ahead of print, 2022 Aug 10]. Arch Orthop Trauma Surg 2022. https://doi.org/10.1007/s00402-022-04574-3.
37. Stake IK, Ræder BW, Gregersen MG, et al. Higher complication rate after nail compared with plate fixation of ankle fractures in patients aged 60 years or older: a prospective, randomized controlled trial. Bone Joint Lett J 2023;105-B(1): 72–81.
38. Ayoub MA. Ankle fractures in diabetic neuropathic arthropathy: can tibiotalar arthrodesis salvage the limb? J Bone Joint Surg Br 2008;90(7):906–14.
39. Ebaugh MP, Umbel B, Goss D, et al. Outcomes of primary tibiotalocalcaneal nailing for complicated diabetic ankle fractures. Foot Ankle Int 2019;40(12):1382–7.
40. Bazarov I, Peace RA, Lagaay PM, et al. Early protected weightbearing after ankle fractures in patients with diabetes mellitus. J Foot Ankle Surg 2017;56(1):30–3.
41. Olsen JR, Hunter J, Baumhauer JF. Osteoporotic ankle fractures. Orthop Clin North Am 2013;44(2):225–41.
42. Black DM, Cummings SR, Karpf DB, et al. Randomised trial of effect of alendronate on risk of fracture in women with existing vertebral fractures. Fracture Intervention Trial Research Group. Lancet 1996;348(9041):1535–41.

43. Harris ST, Watts NB, Genant HK, et al. Effects of risedronate treatment on verte-bral and nonvertebral fractures in women with postmenopausal osteoporosis: a randomized controlled trial. Vertebral Efficacy with Risedronate Therapy (VERT) Study Group. JAMA 1999;282(14):1344–52.
44. McClung MR, Geusens P, Miller PD, et al. Effect of risedronate on the risk of hip fracture in elderly women. Hip Intervention Program Study Group. N Engl J Med 2001;344(5):333–40.
45. LeBoff MS, Chou SH, Ratliff KA, et al. Supplemental vitamin D and incident frac-tures in midlife and older adults. N Engl J Med 2022;387(4):299–309.

Considerations with Fractures of the Posterior Malleolus in Ankle Fractures

Jason D. Pollard, DPM, FACFAS[a],*, Craig E. Krcal Jr, DPM[b,c]

KEYWORDS

- Ankle fracture • Classification • Fracture • Posterior lateral approach
- Posterior medial approach • Surgery

KEY POINTS

- Lateral radiographs of trimalleolar ankle fractures fail to accurately demonstrate the size, articular involvement, and presence of possible die-punch fragments of posterior malleolar fractures. There should be a low threshold for obtaining a post-reduction 3D CT scan to more precisely access the fracture pattern and aid in surgical planning.
- Posterior malleolar fractures with a medial extension (Haraguchi Type II) tend to have a poorer prognosis as compared to those without.
- Direct fixation of posterior malleolus fracture, through a posterior medial or posterior lateral approach, has been shown to have a lower mal-reduction rate as compared to indirect fixation with anterior to posterior screw fixation.
- Anatomic reduction and direct fracture stabilization of the posterior malleolus provide greater stabilization to the syndesmosis as compared to trans-syndesmotic fixation.

INTRODUCTION

Ankle fractures are among the most common orthopedic injuries, accounting for up to 10% of all osseous injuries, and this incidence is expected to uptrend over the next few decades with a rise in the aging population. Epidemiologically, literature has shown between 15 and 40% of ankle fractures to be trimalleolar in nature with isolated posterior malleolar fractures alone encompassing less than 5% of ankle fractures. Elderly individuals, particularly females between 60 and 69 years of age have shown to be more vulnerable to trimalleolar ankle fractures.[1,2] Trimalleolar ankle fractures can vary in pathomechanics from low energy rotational injuries to axially loaded

[a] Department of Podiatric Surgery, Kaiser Permanente, 3600 Broadway, Suite 17, Oakland, CA 94611, USA; [b] The CORE Institute, 18444 North 25th Avenue Suite 320, Phoenix, AZ 85023, USA; [c] Graduate Kaiser San Francisco Bay Area Foot & Ankle Residency, 2023
* Corresponding author.
E-mail address: Jason.pollard@kp.org

moderate to high energy pilon-type fractures, with the former accounting for nearly two-thirds of trimalleolar ankle fractures.[3,4]

There is ample literature to support the operative management of trimalleolar ankle fractures due to their inherent instability. Non-operative management, even in the setting of appropriate analgesia, reduction and close contact casting, can be remarkably difficult to maintain reduction, resulting in subsequent malunion and rapid progression to post-traumatic arthritis and deformity.[5–9] Interestingly, although the operative management of trimalleolar ankle fractures is widely accepted, there is still great debate when it comes to the management of the posterior colliculus. There have been no validated criteria to determine which the posterior malleolus (PM) should be directly or indirectly fixed.

Historically, the size of the PM fracture has guided decision-making as to when to fix the posterior malleolus.[5–10] A plethora of cadaveric studies have set out to identify the implications of posterior malleolar fractures as they relate to the alteration of contact pressure of the tibiotalar joint. Macko and colleagues[11] insinuated predictable accelerated post traumatic arthritis in their cadaveric model when the size of the posterior malleolus fracture involved 25% or more of the articular surface of the tibia due to changes in contact pressure. Similarly, Hartford and coworkers created posterior malleolar fractures in cadaveric specimens involving 25%, 33%, and 50% of the articular surface measured on lateral ankle radiographs, and they found a corresponding decrease of tibiotalar contact area with increasing fracture fragment size of 4%, 13% and 22%, respectively. They concluded that a statistically significant decrease in tibiotalar contact area can be expected with fracture fragments involving more than 33% of the tibiotalar joint.[12] In contrast, Vrahas and colleagues[13] evaluated the change in peak pressure when removing roughly 40% of the posterior malleolus using a static axial loaded cadaveric ankle model and noted no change in peak pressure throughout the tibiotalar joint as compared with uninjured ankles. Fitzpatrick and colleagues[14] took this study one step further and looked at dynamic loading of the ankle through dorsiflexion and plantarflexion range of motion with the removal of 50% of the posterior malleolus, ultimately concluding there was no significant increase in peak pressures, but rather the redistribution of load to the central and anterior tibiotalar joint. Needless to say, there remains significant debate in the literature regarding a "size" cutoff in when to fix posterior malleolus fractures.

On the other hand, there are evolving views as to the role the posterior malleolus contribute to ankle joint stability. Frequently, trimalleolar ankle fractures are amenable to open reduction and internal fixation of the medial and lateral malleolus with or without the use of trans-syndesmotic fixation; this incarcerates the talus in the ankle joint mortise. This technique is often times enough to restore and maintain a stable ankle joint mortise.[15] Recent cadaveric studies have suggested ankle joint instability when there is loss of the posterior constraint of the ankle joint, especially in combination with a compromised lateral buttress as seen with Weber B or Weber C fibular fractures.[16] Finally, there has been an increasing body of literature that notes the inherent risk and morbidity in the use of trans-syndesmotic fixation with discrepancies in reduction techniques, fixation, and an alarmingly high syndesmotic malreduction rates verified on postoperative CT scans as high as 52%.[17–20]

A deep understanding of ankle joint anatomy is needed to discern which structures are compromised, opposed to those uninjured with these complex fracture patterns. The syndesmosis, more specifically, the posterior inferior tibiofibular ligament (PITFL) has been a topic of much research following the landmark article by Ogilvie-Harris in which the PITFL was found to account for 42% of syndesmotic stability in his cadaveric model.[21] This is relevant to the posterior malleolus fracture topic, as a fracture of the posterior malleolus (Volkman's fracture), by definition, implies some degree of compromise to syndesmotic stability. This has led many authors and practitioners to pursue anatomic reduction of the posterior malleolus, independent of size, to allow anatomic restoration of the physiologic tension of the PITFL.[22–24]

These factors may play a role in patient outcomes when considering posterior malleolar fractures and the etiology of posttraumatic arthritis. It is widely accepted that articular congruity plays a significant role in predicting posttraumatic arthritis, however predicting posttraumatic arthritis following ankle ORIF is much less predictable with arthritis rates around 30%.[24–26] At this time, however, long term data is not available to reliably predict these outcomes of these patients. Furthermore, the role of the posterior malleolus plays in the advancement of posttraumatic arthritis is unclear.

PATHOANATOMY OF POSTERIOR MALLEOLUS FRACTURE

The osseous structures which comprise the distal tibia include the medial malleolus, posterior malleolus and tibial incisura. The PM serves as the tibial attachment site of the posterior inferior tibio-fibular ligament (PITFL), which has been shown in previous cadaveric studies to contribute up to 42% of the distal tibiofibular syndesmosis stability.[21] Gardner and colleagues found that on the MRI evaluation of acute PER IV ankle fractures involving PM fractures, the PITFL remains intact to its distal tibial attachment. They further concluded in a cadaveric model that the fixation of the PM fracture restored 70% of stiffness of the syndesmosis as compared to transmalleolar screw stabilization, which only offered 40% restoration when compared to intact specimens.[22,27]

Posterior malleolar fracture morphology has also been shown to determine outcomes in rotational ankle fractures. Blom and colleagues[27] found that fractures of the PM with a medial extension (Haraguchi Type II) are associated with poorer functional outcomes as compared to those without a medial extension (Haraguchi Type I and Type III). Therefore, PM fracture size should not be the only indication to address PM fractures, but also fracture morphology, displacement, articular incongruity/impaction and syndesmotic instability. Bartoníček and colleagues[28] further defined PM fracture on the presence or absence of incisura involvement on CT and 3D CT scans and proposed a classification scheme based on these findings. They concluded that the fixation and stabilization of PM fractures not only restores the articular surface of the distal tibia, but also the integrity of the fibular notch. Inappropriate reduction of the PM and subsequently the fibular notch, may result in a symptomatic mal-union and progressive post-traumatic arthritis of the ankle joint.

In addition to PM fracture size, other investigations have examined the importance of fracture height. Wang and coworkers noted a positive correlation between fracture height and fracture area. They also found that PM fractures with "die-punch" lesions also tended to have a greater average height than those without.[29]

EVALUATION/IMAGING/CLASSIFICATION

Clinical evaluation of ankle fractures with PM involvement should be thorough but focused. The assessment of the neurovascular bundle along with myotendinous structures and ligamentous constraints supporting the ankle joint should be completed. Obvious ankle joint instability may be present along with deformity and skin tenting, all of which should be addressed as quickly as possible with appropriate closed reduction and splinting. Ankle fractures involving a large posterior malleolar component can be particularly difficult to maintain a closed reduction as the posterior constraint of the ankle joint no longer prevents the talus from posterior subluxation or dislocation. In our experience, a well-padded plaster of paris splint with the ankle held in slight plantarflexion can keep the talus beneath the tibia and hold the PM fracture reduced as this prevents the ankle joint capsule from tightening and displacing the posterior constraint. If the talus continues to sublux or dislocate posteriorly at the ankle mortise despite adequate closed reduction and splinting, then acute surgical stabilization may be required with either definitive ORIF or temporary external fixation as dictated by the soft tissue envelope.

Plain film radiographs are standard for the initial evaluation of ankle fractures, however, an appropriate, orthogonal lateral projection of the ankle joint with a molded splint will many times fail to demonstrate the true size or extent of articular involvement of a PM fracture. This is oftentimes due to either poor image quality from the overlying split material which may obscure any die-punch type lesions or an inadequate projection of the ankle joint or posterior malleolus fracture line which usually underestimates the size of the PM fracture and amount of intraarticular extension.

Two studies highlight just how difficult and deceiving an accurate estimation of PM size and intraarticular involvement can be. Meijer and colleagues undertook a study where 100 orthopedic trauma surgeons review 31 trimalleolar ankle fractures with lateral projection plain films to estimate the size of a posterior malleolar fracture as a percentage of the tibial plafond surface, with a follow up question of whether they would fix the posterior malleolus fracture. The average posterior malleolar observer estimation of fragment size was 24.4% of the plafond. The actual average posterior malleolar fragment involved only 13.5% as measured on quantitative 3D-CT scanning. The result was a diagnostic accuracy of just 22% with an interobserver agreement of 0.61.[30]

Kumar and colleagues aimed to look at the effect a CT scan might have on operative planning as it pertains to malleolar fractures. Three observers prospectively studied 56 consecutive malleolar ankle fractures. An operative plan was first made using plain film radiographs alone, each observer subsequently created a preoperative plan with the associated CT scan. In 23.2% of cases, the operative plan changed following the assessment of the CT scan with the most common indication being an underappreciation of the morphology of the PM fracture.[31]

These studies along with the aforementioned difficulties in assessing PM fractures with plain film radiographs suggest that we should obtain CT scans in most PM fractures. Once a CT scan is obtained, the surgeon must then be able to decipher the proper surgical approach and method by which to stabilize the fractures. There are multiple classifications which aim to provide diagnostic and prognostic value to fractures involving the posterior malleolus, including: Haraguchi, and Bartonicek & Rammelt.[3,4]

The most referred to classification is the Haraguchi classification. This landmark article set out to define the pathoanatomy of posterior malleolar fractures after retrospectively reviewing CT scans and mapping fracture patterns in 57 consecutive patients with posterior malleolar fractures. Haraguchi and colleagues[3] identified three posterior malleolar fracture types, ultimately stating that fracture lines are highly variable and the routine use of CT scans in this patient population should be considered as 20% of the posterior malleolar fractures had medial malleolar extension which could not easily be identified on plain films. This idea is again supported by the Bartonicek and Rammelt classification which identified 5 subgroups of posterior malleolar fractures again placing emphasis on the importance of CT scans to appropriately identify not only the intraarticular extent of posterior malleolar fractures and medial malleolar involvement, but also to identify extension into the fibular incisura which may clue us into the overall stability and reducibility of the tibiotalar joint.[4] Although each classification set out to identify fracture patterns and treatment options for each, they fall short in providing prognostic value compared with other lower extremity classifications.

SURGICAL TECHNIQUE
Posterior Lateral Approach

Following general or spinal anesthesia the patient is placed onto a radiolucent operating table in a prone position with the feet just extending beyond the end of the operating room table. A thigh tourniquet can be placed for hemostasis and all bony prominences should be well padded and axillary support should be utilized to avoid abdominal compression and to allow for unimpeded chest wall movement (**Fig. 1**A). The C-arm should be placed on the contralateral side of the injury and perpendicular to the operative extremity (**Fig. 1**B). This will allow for unobstructed AP and mortise views of the ankle, as well as a cross table lateral radiograph with the use of appropriate sterile draping.

The incision is placed mid-line between the lateral border of the Achilles tendon and peroneal tendons (**Fig. 2**). Care should be taken to identify and protect the sural nerve throughout the procedure (**Fig. 3**). Next the talocrural fascia is incised parallel to the incision exposing the flexor hallucis longus (FHL) muscle belly (**Fig. 4**A). The FHL is retracted medially along with the neurovascular bundle exposing the PM fracture (**Fig. 4**B). The fracture is irrigated and evacuated of any hematoma and any intercalary fragments can be addressed as needed. It is the senior author's preference to then expose, reduce and provisionally clamp the lateral malleolus fracture at this time, as the PM is still tethered to the lateral malleolus through the PITFL (**Fig. 5**A–C). Failure

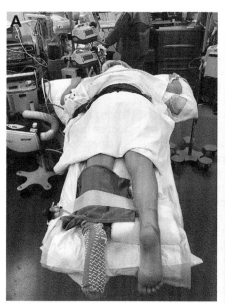
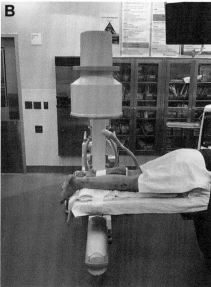

Fig. 1. (*A*) Prone positioning for posterior malleolus open reduction and internal fixation (ORIF). A radiolucent table should be utilized with the foot hanging just off the edge of the table and all bony prominence padded and airway protected. (*B*) C-arm should be placed on the contralateral side and perpendicular to the lower extremity. This will allow for AP and mortise views of the ankle. Cross table lateral radiograph can be completed by flexing the operative knee and use of sterile draping.

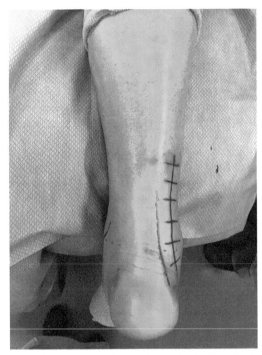

Fig. 2. Incision placement for a posterior lateral ORIF. The incision is placed between the interval of the lateral border of the Achilles tendon and the peroneal tendons.

to first restore the fibula length and rotation may impede the anatomic reduction of the PM fracture. Plating of the lateral malleolus should not be performed at this time, as this can impede the radiographic visualization of the PM on lateral radiographs. If any medial malleolus fracture is present, then a medial incision is performed, and the fracture should be anatomically reduced and provisionally pinned. The reason to reduce the medial malleolus fracture at this time is again for the concern that the definitive fixation of the PM fracture prior to any medial fracture reduction could potentially impede anatomic reduction for those PM fractures with a medial extension (Haraguchi Type II). Once the lateral malleolus, and if present medial malleolus fracture, have been reduced and provisionally stabilized, then the PM fracture can be fixated with either lag screws or an under contoured one-third tubular anti-glide plate and/or specialty PM plate as the fracture pattern may dictate (**Fig. 6**A–C). If there is any difficulty with PM fracture reduction, a large bone reduction forceps may be utilized to help reduce the fracture (**Fig. 7**). Next attention can be directed to the lateral and medial malleolus fractures for definitive fixation (**Fig. 8**).

Following the stabilization of all fractures, an intra-operative stress exam of the syndesmosis should be performed. If any syndesmotic instability is noted, then stabilization can be performed as needed with either a trans-syndesmotic screw or a flexible syndesmotic fixation device. The incision is then irrigated and closed in a layer fashion (**Fig. 9**) and an appropriate post-operative splint applied.

Posterior Medial Approach

For patients with a two-part PM fracture with a medial extension (Haraguchi Type II/ Bartonicek & Rammelt Type 3), or for those with an associated medial malleolus/

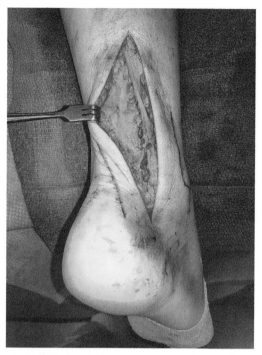

Fig. 3. Care should be taken to identify and protect the sural nerve throughout the procedure.

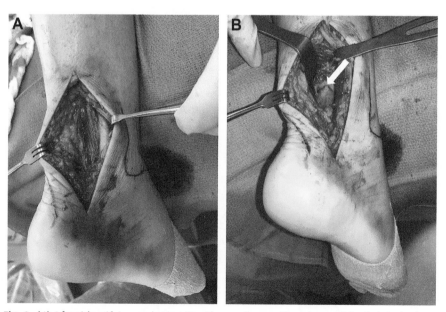

Fig. 4. (*A*) After identifying and retracting the sural nerve the talocrural fascia is incised parallel with the incision exposing the flexor hallucis longus (FHL) muscle belly. (*B*) The FHL tendon, along with the neurovascular bundle is retracted medially exposing the PM fracture. (*White arrow* notes apex of posterior malleolus fracture).

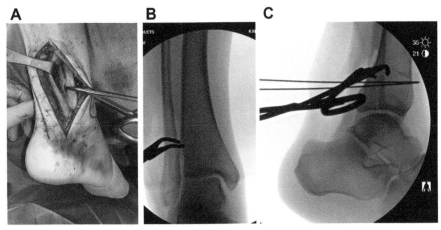

Fig. 5. (*A*) The peroneal tendons are retracted medially exposing the lateral malleolus fracture. The lateral malleolus fracture is reduced and temporarily clamped with a bone reduction forceps or lobster claw. Plating the lateral malleolus fracture should be avoided at this time, as it will impede subsequent lateral ankle radiographs to evaluated for PM reduction. (*B*) AP radiographs following lateral malleolus fracture reduction with the restoration of fibular length and rotation. (*C*) Lateral radiograph demonstrating lateral malleolus fracture reduction with the reduction and pinning of the PM fracture.

anterior colliculus fracture, a posterior medial approach can be performed (**Fig. 10**). Following standard open reduction and internal fixation of the lateral malleolus fracture, a medial incision is fashioned which follows the posterior medial border of the distal tibia and extends anteriorly at its distal aspect. Care is taken to identify the saphenous vein and nerve which are retracted anteriorly. The flexor retinaculum is then incised exposing the flexor tendons. The tendon sheath of the posterior tibial tendon is incised and the interval between the posterior tibial tendon and flexor digitorum longus (FDL) tendon is developed to expose the fracture. The posterior tibial

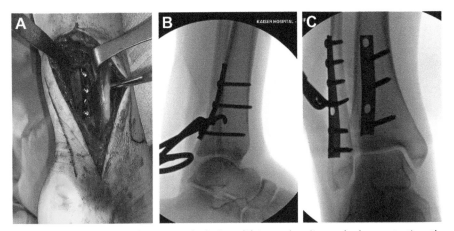

Fig. 6. (*A*) PM fracture reduction and plating. (*B*) Lateral radiograph demonstrating the anatomic reduction and internal fixation of PM fracture with a 1/3 tubular anti-glade plate. (*C*) Mortise radiograph following ORIF of a posterior and lateral malleolus fracture.

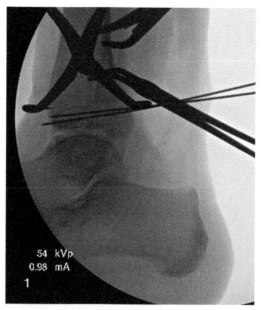

Fig. 7. Large reduction bone forceps to help reduce and compress PM fracture.

tendon is retracted anteriorly, while the FDL and neurovascular bundle are retracted posteriorly. The fracture is then evacuated of any hematoma, anatomically reduced, and fixated depending on the nature and orientation of the medial fracture pattern (**Fig. 11**).

CLINICAL OUTCOMES

Treatment approaches have evolved over the last few decades in an attempt to improve outcomes of trimalleolar ankle fractures. There have been no randomized

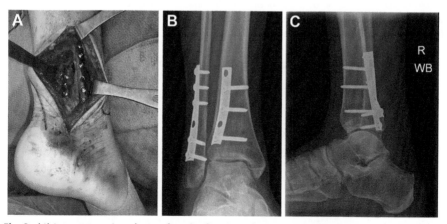

Fig. 8. (*A*) Intra-operative photo after the fixation of posterior malleolus and lateral malleolus fractures. (*B*) Final weight bearing mortise radiograph of the ankle. (*C*) Final weight bearing lateral radiograph of the ankle following ORIF bi-malleolar ankle fracture.

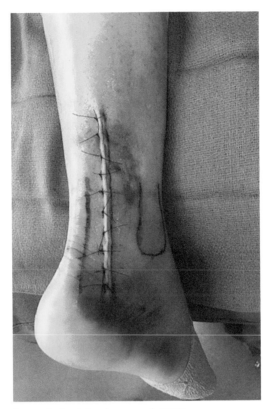

Fig. 9. Skin closure for posterior lateral approach ORIF.

controlled trials that have found predictive factors regarding outcomes in trimalleolar ankle fractures, but the general consensus in providing these patients with the best outcome is anatomic reduction and appropriate stabilization of the ankle joint. When to pursue fixation of the posterior malleolus, and how to do so remains controversial, though there is an increasing body of literature that would support the routine fixation of most posterior malleolar fractures.[32–35]

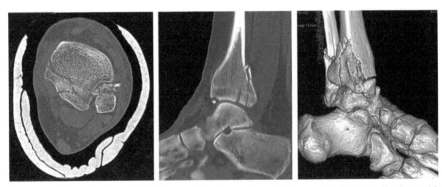

Fig. 10. Axial, sagittal and 3D-CT scan of a two-part posterior malleolus trimalleolar ankle fracture.

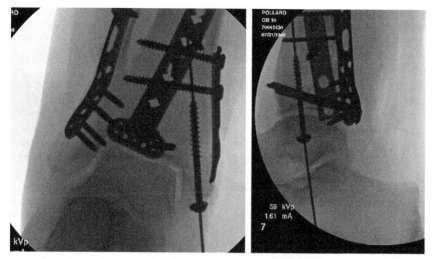

Fig. 11. Intra-operative mortise and lateral radiographs following ORIF via a lateral and posterior medial approach of a two-part posterior malleolus trimalleolar ankle fracture.

Saad and colleagues retrospectively looked at 117 trimalleolar or trimalleolar equivalent ankle fractures with direct posterior malleolar fixation and indirect fixation–defined as direct reduction and fixation or indirect fixation via fixation of medial and lateral malleolus with syndesmotic stabilization. The average cut off size of the posterior malleolus direct fixation group was roughly 25% of the tibiotalar joint articulation. They aimed to look at short term outcomes via PROMIS scores of each cohort and found no difference in total pain and total function between the 2 groups. However, this data may be difficult to extrapolate to clinical applications due to the short follow-up period and lack of identification of injury pattern, energy, and posterior malleolar classification.[35]

Shi and colleagues[36] compared direct posterior lateral approach (n = 64) to indirect (anterior to posterior screws) (n = 52) reduction of posterior malleolar fractures in patients with >25% of tibiotalar articular involvement and found the quality of reduction to be superior in direct reduction and fixation group via evaluation of postoperative CT scans, as well as improved AOFAS scores with no difference in range of motion or VAS scores.

Over the last few decades, there has been a mounting body of literature to support the fixation of smaller posterior malleolar fracture fragments as it pertains to trimalleolar ankle fractures in an attempt to restore true plafond morphology along with, arguably more importantly, tibiotalar joint stability with native ligamentous tension. Verhage and colleagues published on 169 retrospectively fixed trimalleolar ankle fractures at a level 1 trauma center with a respectable follow-up of mean 6.3 years. Average fragment size was 17% with 23% of these patients' undergoing the fixation of the PM. Though clinical union was found in all 169 patients on follow-up, they found a persistent step off larger than 1 mm to be an independent, significant risk factor for the development of osteoarthritis along with increased age. AOFAS functional outcomes were worse in patients with evidence of OA and increased BMI.[37]

Miller and colleagues looked at the stability of the syndesmosis following ankle ORIF with and without direct posterior malleolar fracture fixation. A total of 198 patients were evaluated, of which 76.3% (N = 151) were initially positioned supine, while 23.7% (N = 47) were initially positioned prone. In the group of patients initially positioned supine, 48.3% needed some form of additional stabilization with either indirect fixation of the PM fracture and/or trans-syndemotic screw fixation. By contrast only 2.1% of patients who were placed prone and underwent direct fixation of the PM fracture needed additional syndesmotic stabilization. This resulted in a 13-fold higher syndesmotic instability rate observed in the supine group (P < .001).[15] This is significant when considering the aforementioned malreduction rates when looking at transyndesmotic fixation.

Finally, in a retrospective study by Yang and colleagues, 113 patients with bimalleolar or trimalleolar ankle fractures with syndesmotic injury and at least 24 months follow-up were evaluated following ORIF with syndesmotic screw stabilization. Of the 3 groups in this study (I = bimalleolar, II = trimalleolar fracture with syndesmotic screw removal at 6–8 weeks and III = trimalleolar fracture with screw removal at 3 months), they found early syndesmotic screw removal (Group II) to correlate with residual syndesmosis instability at a rate of nearly 21%. This may support the fixation of even smaller posterior malleolar fracture to appropriately restore the stability of the tibiotalar joint and distal syndesmosis.[38]

The advancement of outcomes pertaining to posterior malleolar fractures in the setting of trimalleolar ankle fractures will require further, stronger powered research with long term outcomes to assess the potential benefits or drawbacks to the fixation of posterior malleolar ankle fractures, regardless of size, with the aim to decrease the incidence of posttraumatic arthritis.

COMPLICATIONS

Though literature evaluating outcomes of the fixation of the posterior malleolus are less concrete, it is well established that the fixation of the posterior malleolus is a safe procedure, including the prone posterior medial and posterior lateral approaches. Obvious concerns include the violation of pertinent posterior neurovascular structures–most notably the posterior neurovascular bundle and the sural nerve. Veltman and colleagues noted a low complication rate in their large systemic review of 886 posterior malleolar fractures who underwent ORIF. They found remarkably low complication rates and need for subsequent surgery with persistent posterior malleolar step off >2 mm less than 4% of the time, post-traumatic arthritis at 44 months of 2%, infection of 2%, hardware removal of 11% and subsequent surgery of 13%.[39] Bali and colleagues specifically looked at the efficacy of the posterior medial approach to Haraguchi Type II PM fractures. Although they did have a small sample size (N = 15), they noted a median Olerud- Molander Ankle Score of 72. A single patient had medial forefoot paraesthesia immediately postoperatively, which resolved within 3 months.[40] Once the neurovascular structures have been identified and safely retracted, the visualization to the posterior tibia is unmatched compared with other approaches. Further, we often place large plates on these injuries, and the posterior leg lends itself to excellent soft tissue coverage compared with the medial and lateral soft tissue envelope. Foot and ankle surgeons who routinely fix ankle fractures should be very familiar and comfortable with these approaches to provide predictable outcomes for these difficult injuries.

CLINICS CARE POINTS

- Trimalleolar ankle fractures have a worse prognosis as compared to unimalleolar or bimalleolar ankle fractures. In addition, PM fractures with a medial extension tend to have poorer outcomes as compared to those PM fractures without a medial extension.

- Plain lateral radiographs of trimalleolar ankle fractures oftentimes fail to accurately depict the size, articular involvement, and possible intercalary fragments of posterior malleolus fractures. It is for these reasons we now have a much lower threshold to obtain a post-reduction 3D-CT scan of the ankle to further assist in surgical planning including the incisional approach and method of fixation.

- Previous studies evaluating post-operative CT scan of PM fracture fixation have shown a lower mal-reduction rate with direct fixation via a posterior lateral approach versus indirect fixation with anterior-posterior screws.[36]

- Greater stiffness is restored to the syndesmosis with the direct fixation of the PM fracture as compared to indirect stabilization with trans-syndesmotic fixation.[12]

- Foot and ankle surgeon should be familiar with both the posterior medial and posterior lateral approach as well as fixation methods of PM fractures. Proper patient positioning, use of a radiolucent table and a well-trained Radiology Technician will aid in obtaining proper orthogonal views of the ankle to accurately assess intra-operatively the reduction of PM fractures.

DISCLOSURE

None.

REFERENCES

1. Pflüger P, Braun KF, Mair O, et al. Current management of trimalleolar ankle fractures. EFORT Open Reviews 2021;6(8):692–703.
2. Koval KJ, Lurie J, Zhou W, et al. Ankle fractures in the elderly. J Orthop Trauma 2005;19(9):635–9.
3. Haraguchi N, Haruyama H, Toga H, et al. Pathoanatomy of posterior malleolar fractures of the ankle. J Bone Joint Surg 2006;88(5):1085–92.
4. Rammelt S, Bartoníček J. Posterior malleolar fractures. JBJS Reviews 2020;8(8). https://doi.org/10.2106/jbjs.rvw.19.00207.
5. McDaniel WJ, Wilson FC. Trimalleolar fractures of the ankle. An end result study. Clin Orthop Relat Res 1977;(122). https://doi.org/10.1097/00003086-197701000-00006.
6. Jaskulka RA, Ittner G, Schedl R. Fractures of the posterior tibial margin. J Trauma Inj Infect Crit Care 1989;29(11):1565–70.
7. Ali MS, McLaren CA, Rouholamin E, et al. Ankle fractures in the elderly: nonoperative or operative treatment. J Orthop Trauma 1987;1(4):275–80.
8. Willett K, Keene DJ, Mistry D, et al. Close contact casting vs surgery for initial treatment of unstable ankle fractures in older adults. JAMA 2016;316(14):1455.
9. Makwana NK, Bhowal B, Harper WM, Hui AW. Conservative versus operative treatment for displaced ankle fractures in patients over 55 years of age. A prospective, randomised study. J Bone Joint Surg Br 2001;83(4):525–9.
10. Gardner MJ, Streubel PN, McCormick JJ, et al. Surgeon practices regarding operative treatment of posterior malleolus fractures. Foot Ankle Int 2011;32(4):385–93.
11. Macko VW, Matthews LS, Zwirkoski P, et al. The joint-contact area of the ankle. the contribution of the posterior malleolus. J Bone Joint Surg 1991;73(3):347–51.
12. Hartford JM, Gorczyca JT, McNamara JL, Mayor MB. Tibiotalar contact area. Contribution of posterior malleolus and deltoid ligament. Clin Orthop Relat Res 1995;320:182–7.

13. Vrahas M, Fu F, Veenis B. Intraarticular contact stresses with simulated ankle malunions. J Orthop Trauma 1994;8(2):159–66.
14. Fitzpatrick DC, Otto JK, McKinley TO, et al. Kinematic and contact stress analysis of posterior malleolus fractures of the ankle. J Orthop Trauma 2004;18(5):271–8.
15. Miller MA, McDonald TC, Graves ML, et al. Stability of syndesmosis after posterior malleolar fracture fixation. Foot Ankle Int 2018;39(1):99–104.
16. Raasch WG, Larkin JJ, Draganich LF. Assessment of the posterior malleolus as a restraint to posterior subluxation of the ankle. J Bone Joint Surg 1992;74(8):1201–6.
17. Boszczyk A, Kwapisz S, Krümmel M, et al. Correlation of incisura anatomy with syndesmotic malreduction. Foot Ankle Int 2017;39(3):369–75.
18. Cherney SM, Spraggs-Hughes AG, McAndrew CM, et al. Incisura morphology as a risk factor for syndesmotic malreduction. Foot Ankle Int 2016;37(7):748–54.
19. Gardner MJ, Demetrakopoulos D, Briggs SM, et al. Malreduction of the tibiofibular syndesmosis in ankle fractures. Foot Ankle Int 2006;27(10):788–92.
20. Cosgrove CT, Putnam SM, Cherney SM, et al. Medial clamp tine positioning affects ankle syndesmosis malreduction. J Orthop Trauma 2017;31(8):440–6.
21. Ogilvie-Harris DJ, Reed SC, Hedman TP. Disruption of the ankle syndesmosis: biomechanical study of the ligamentous restraints. Arthrosc J Arthrosc Relat Surg 1994;10(5):558–60.
22. Gardner MJ, Brodsky A, Briggs SM, et al. Fixation of posterior malleolar fractures provides greater syndesmotic stability. Clin Orthop Relat Res 2006;447:165–71.
23. Behery O, Narayanan R, Konda SR, et al. Posterior malleolar fixation reduces the incidence of trans-syndesmotic fixation in rotational ankle fracture repair. Iowa Orthop J 2021;41(1):121–5.
24. Beak JS, Kim YT, Lee SH. Predisposing factors for posttraumatic osteoarthritis after malleolus fracture fixation in patients younger than 50 years. Foot Ankle Int 2021;43(3):389–97.
25. McHale S, Williams M, Ball T. Retrospective cohort study of operatively treated ankle fractures involving the posterior malleolus. Foot Ankle Surg 2020;26(2):138–45.
26. Gardner MJ, Demetrakopoulos D, Briggs SM, et al. The ability of the lauge-hansen classification to predict ligament injury and mechanism in ankle fractures: an MRI study. J Orthop Trauma 2006;20(4):267–72.
27. Blom RP, Meijer DT, de Muinck Keizer RJO, et al. Posterior malleolar fracture morphology determines outcome in rotational type ankle fractures. Injury 2019;50(7):1392–7.
28. Bartoníček J, Rammelt S, Kostlivý K, et al. Anatomy and classification of the posterior tibial fragment in ankle fractures. Arch Orthop Trauma Surg 2015;135(4):505–16.
29. Wang Z, Yuan C, Zhu G, et al. A retrospective study on the morphology of posterior malleolar fractures based on a CT scan: whether we ignore the importance of fracture height. BioMed Res Int 2020;1–8. https://doi.org/10.1155/2020/2903537.
30. Meijer DT, Doornberg JN, Sierevelt IN, et al. Guesstimation of posterior malleolar fractures on lateral plain radiographs. Injury 2015;46(10):2024–9.
31. Kumar A, Mishra P, Tandon A, et al. Effect of CT on management plan in malleolar ankle fractures. Foot Ankle Int 2017;39(1):59–66.
32. Tejwani NC, Pahk B, Egol KA. Effect of posterior malleolus fracture on outcome after unstable ankle fracture. J Trauma 2010;69:666–9.

33. Mason LW, Kaye A, Widnall J, et al. Posterior malleolar ankle fractures: an effort at improving outcomes. JB JS Open Access 2019;4:e0058.
34. Jeyaseelan L, Bua N, Parker L, et al. Outcomes of posterior malleolar fixation in ankle fractures in a major trauma centre. Injury 2021;52(4):1023–7.
35. Saad BN, Rampertaap Y, Menken LG, et al. Direct versus indirect posterior malleolar fixation in the treatment of trimalleolar ankle fractures: is there a difference in outcomes? OTA International: The Open Access Journal of Orthopaedic Trauma 2022;5(4). https://doi.org/10.1097/oi9.0000000000000219.
36. Shi H-fei, Xiong J, Chen YX, et al. Comparison of the direct and indirect reduction techniques during the surgical management of posterior malleolar fractures. BMC Muscoskel Disord 2017;18(1). https://doi.org/10.1186/s12891-017-1475-7.
37. Verhage SM, Krijnen P, Schipper IB, et al. Persistent postoperative step-off of the posterior malleolus leads to higher incidence of post-traumatic osteoarthritis in trimalleolar fractures. Arch Orthop Trauma Surg 2018;139(3):323–9.
38. Yang T-C, Tzeng YH, Wang CS, et al. Untreated small posterior fragment of ankle fracture with early removal of syndesmotic screw is associated with recurrent syndesmotic instability. Injury 2021;52(3):638–43.
39. Veltman ES, Halma JJ, de Gast A. Longterm outcome of 886 posterior malleolar fractures: a systematic review of the literature. Foot Ankle Surg 2016;22(2):73–7.
40. Bali N, Aktselis I, Ramasamy A, et al. An evolution in the management of fractures of the ankle. The Bone & Joint Journal 2017;99-B(11):1496–501.

Navigating the Challenges of Total Ankle Replacement
Deformity Correction and Infection Considerations

Joseph D. Dickinson, DPM[a], David R. Collman, DPM[b],
Lindsay H. Russel, DPM[c], Danny J. Choung, DPM[d],*

KEYWORDS

- Ankle arthritis • Varus • Valgus ankle deformity • Ankle periprosthetic joint infection

KEY POINTS

- Total ankle replacement demands significant technical expertise and precision. It is a complex and nuanced operation with a steep learning curve.
- The successful correction of end-stage ankle arthritis with significant coronal deformity requires a thoughtful patient selection process, a methodical approach to the implementation of ancillary procedures, and adaptability in surgical techniques. These strategies are essential to achieve comprehensive deformity correction and optimal prosthetic alignment to promote functional outcomes and durability of the prosthesis.
- Periprosthetic infection in total ankle replacement is challenging to diagnose and treat because of biofilm and unforgiving soft tissues. The risk of failure in single-stage treatment may be unacceptably high.

INTRODUCTION

Ankle arthritis in its advanced stage presents several similarities with other degenerative weight-bearing joint disorders affecting the lower limbs. Consequently, it inflicts

[a] Kaiser San Francisco Bay Area Foot and Ankle Residency Program, Department of Orthopedics/Podiatry, Kaiser Permanente Oakland Medical Center, 3600 Broadway, Oakland, CA 94611, USA; [b] Kaiser San Francisco Bay Area Foot and Ankle Residency Program, Department of Orthopedics, Podiatry, Injury, Sports Medicine, Kaiser Permanente San Francisco Medical Center, 4506th Avenue, French Campus, 5th Floor, San Francisco, CA 94118, USA; [c] Department of Orthopedics, Kaiser Permanente South Sacramento Medical Center, 6600 Bruceville Road, Sacramento, CA 95823, USA; [d] Kaiser North Bay Consortium Foot and Ankle Residency Program, Department of Orthopedics/Podiatry, Kaiser Permanente San Rafael, 99 Montecillo Road, San Rafael, CA 94903, USA
* Corresponding author. Department of Podiatry/Foot and Ankle Surgery, Medical Office Building 2, 2nd Floor, 99 Montecillo Road, San Rafael, CA 94903
E-mail address: danny.choung@kp.org

Clin Podiatr Med Surg 41 (2024) 119–139
https://doi.org/10.1016/j.cpm.2023.06.004
0891-8422/24/© 2023 Elsevier Inc. All rights reserved.

comparable adverse symptoms in patients, including chronic pain, reduced physical capacity, and a substantial decline in their overall health and quality of life. These symptoms closely resemble those reported by individuals with hip[1] or knee arthritis, and the level of physical impairment has been shown to be on par with that of end-stage renal disease and congestive heart failure.[2] In contrast to hip and knee arthritis, end-stage ankle arthritis is primarily caused by previous trauma to the ankle or lower leg, which can impair the structural integrity of the joint and significantly alter its mechanical function and stability. Unfortunately, it often plagues the younger active patient, posing significant challenges, particularly when contemplating total ankle replacement (TAR) while aiming for optimal prosthetic longevity. Furthermore, end-stage ankle arthritis can be complicated by the presence of tibio-talar deformities, which can arise from highly variable conditions affecting joint anatomy or function. Varus and valgus deformities are prevalent in ankle arthritis and can result from various pre-existing conditions such as ligamentous insufficiency, previous intra-articular fractures, fracture malunions, muscle imbalance, significant hindfoot deformity, congenital deformities, and post-traumatic avascular necrosis.

In recent years, TAR has emerged as a rapidly advancing surgical intervention for the management of end-stage ankle arthritis. Favorable outcomes associated with modern advancements in implant design and optimization of surgical instrumentation and technique have propelled the resurgence of this treatment option, which has surpassed the limitations and drawbacks of the first iteration of TAR that was introduced in the 1970s. A comprehensive analysis of the medical literature over the past 2 decades has shown that TAR is an acceptable and increasingly favored alternative to ankle arthrodesis, which was previously regarded as the gold standard surgical procedure for the management of end-stage ankle arthritis. The shift toward TAR is due to concerns associated with subsequent adjacent joint arthritis[3] that have been reported following ankle arthrodesis.

TAR is a complex surgical procedure that requires a high degree of technical skill and experience, arguably surpassing that of ankle arthrodesis in some cases, given the specialized instrumentation and multiple steps involved. The steep learning curve for this procedure demands a high level of accuracy and precision, along with proficient use of the C-arm for appropriate alignment and implant sizing. The distinct biomechanical properties of the ankle joint, coupled with the intricate nature of surgical exposure, contribute to the complexities of TAR. The mechanics of the ankle can be substantially affected by soft tissue insufficiencies or imbalances, as well as by articular or extra-articular structural anomalies, thereby posing formidable obstacles to achieve optimal implant placement, balance, and stability. Even seemingly uncomplicated ankle arthritis cases with a congruent joint can prove to be problematic for surgeons, as they must be capable of detecting subtle nuances that may have gone unnoticed during the preoperative evaluation. Such nuances could include subtle varus bowing of the distal tibia or rotational adaptation of the joint. Failure to account for such factors can potentially result in adverse mechanical imbalance to the prosthesis and thereby compromise its structural integrity. Furthermore, TAR is associated with a higher complication rate compared to other ankle surgeries, and surgeons must be able to identify and manage complications, such as implant loosening, bone cyst formation, or infection, in a timely and effective manner.

The learning curve for TAR surgery can vary depending on the surgeon's level of experience, the type of implant used, and the surgical technique. Additionally, TAR may not be suitable for all patients, and the decision to perform the surgery should be based on a thorough evaluation and discussion of the potential risks and benefits of the procedure.

The advantages of working within a self-contained health care system such as Kaiser Permanente are manifold for foot and ankle surgeons who perform TAR surgery. One of the largest and most comprehensive health care networks in the United States, Kaiser Permanente serves a diverse patient population, which affords its foot and ankle surgeons exposure to a substantial number of patients with end-stage ankle arthritis. Furthermore, this patient population is marked by clinical heterogeneity, often with numerous comorbidities, presenting wide variations in the severity and complexity of ankle arthritis that demand the surgeon's acumen, creativity, preparation, and versatility. A TAR practice in Kaiser Permanente fosters the foot and ankle surgeon's proficiency and enhances their clinical outcomes. This is particularly crucial given the heightened technical challenges associated with coronal plane deformities, which have been more widely acknowledged. However, the integrated care model of Kaiser Permanente presents unique opportunities for collaborative problem-solving with fellow TAR surgeons, effectively sharing knowledge and experience, as well as facilitating important proctoring and mentoring opportunities.

The Neutral Ankle

Mastering the technique in the neutral ankle is essential and fundamental to successfully ascend the learning curve of TAR surgery. In the medical literature, ankles with less than 10° of coronal plane deformity are commonly referred to as having neutral alignment. Although this definition does not denote a completely "normal" ankle joint alignment, it is a useful guideline when considering ancillary procedures that help balance the ankle prosthesis. Modern implant systems incorporate cutting guides and jigs to facilitate alignment of the mechanical axis of the lower extremity. Yet, it is at the discretion and acumen of the surgeon to exercise precision when utilizing these systems to obtain appropriate alignment relative to the several basic planes of the anatomy. In the process of following a stepwise surgical approach to address a debilitating condition, it may become necessary to identify certain contingent anomalies and make necessary adjustments to ensure the integrity of the final outcome. One such phenomenon is the presence of subchondral cysts, which may be detected either prior to or during the procedure. To address this issue, the surgeon may use the resected bone as an autogenous graft to pack the cysts, supplementing with allograft bone as necessary. Properly packing these defects is of utmost importance since they can have a significant impact on the overall stability of the components.

Proficiency with intraoperative fluoroscopy is required for accurate and expeditious positioning of the jigs and cutting guides. The coronal plane should be within 5° of perpendicular to the mechanical axis of the lower extremity. Deviations greater than 5° have been shown to cause increase in local contact pressures by up to 158% and may contribute to bone injury as well as premature polyethylene wear leading to implant failure.[4,5] The angle of the implant in the sagittal plane or "slope" is generally 90° to the mechanical axis. An open slope is typically considered anything less than 90° to the mechanical axis of the lower extremity, which can impact the position of the foot by displacing it anteriorly relative to the tibia. This approach may be used to address or accommodate for certain sagittal based deformities (**Fig. 1**). Conversely, a closed slope is an angle greater than 90° to the mechanical axis and will posteriorly displace the foot relative to the tibia (**Fig. 2**).[6] For the neutral ankle, a perpendicular or slightly open slope is preferred. Axial alignment or rotation of the implant is typically determined using the medial gutter as a reference. However, some literature questions this marker. One study involving 157 arthritic ankles compared medial gutter line versus a line perpendicular to the transmalleolar axis, and found that 51% of the time, these values differed by more than 5°.[7] The implications of this difference

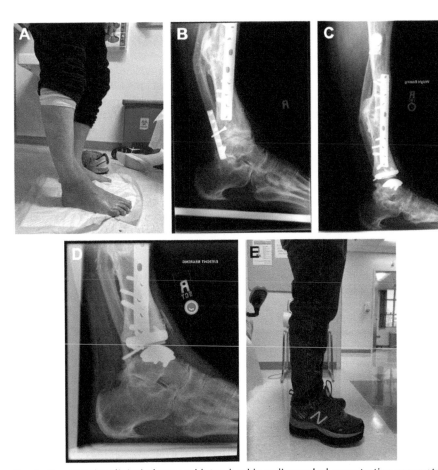

Fig. 1. Preoperative clinical photo and lateral ankle radiograph demonstrating recurvatum malunion of previous tibial fracture, resulting in open slope of the tibial mortise relative to the true anatomic axis (A, B). Postoperative lateral radiographs taken post 6 months and 1 year after surgery demonstrating open slope alignment of the tibial tray to accommodate for the adaptive joint changes related to the tibial malunion (C, D). One year postoperative clinical photo demonstrating improved standing posture with full-length shoe lift to accommodate for the post-traumatic limb-length discrepancy (E).

have yet to be determined clinically, and the medial gutter remains the reference for most of the modern implant systems. In the arthritic ankle, the transmalleolar axis may have adapted to varying degrees of external rotation, necessitating corresponding adjustments to the tibial component orientation at the surgeon's discretion, to minimize any axial anomalies. It is important to remember the foot and talus position when determining alignment. It is recommended to keep the tibial and talar cuts "coupled" to ensure that the tibial and talar components are aligned. "Uncoupled" cuts may be useful and necessary for deformity correction but often demands a higher level of technical expertise. Once the osteotomies are completed, sizing of the implant can begin. It is important to maximize tibial coverage and centralize the talar component. If difficulties arise with seating the tibial trial, it may be necessary to notch either the medial or lateral malleolus, effectively creating more space for the trial, while exercising caution to avoid malleolar fractures. In the event of a malleolar fracture,

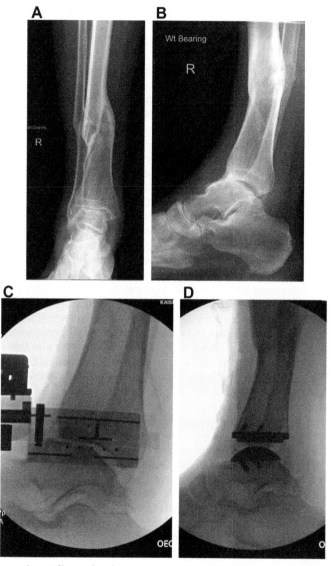

Fig. 2. Preoperative radiographs demonstrate ankle arthritis with malunion of previous tibia-fibula fracture with recurvatum as primary deformity. Note the anterior talar displacement from the mortise on the lateral view (*A, B*). Intraoperative C-arm images depicting closed slope alignment relative to the natural mortise to position the tibial implant in a more neutral position relative to the mechanical axis (*C, D*).

stabilization is imperative to prevent implant instability. The talar trial should cover the talar body without overcrowding the medial and lateral gutters. It is also important to simultaneously align the talar trial to the tibial component while centralizing on the talar body. It has been shown either anterior or posterior malalignment can not only alter ankle range of motion but also the foot bone kinematics and plantar pressures.[8] Furthermore, 5° of sagittal plane malposition can have negative impact to implant function and survivorship.[9] After the components have been properly inserted, polyethylene sizing is the final step for determining appropriate range of motion while maintaining stability.

Coronal Deformities

Ankle arthritis associated with coronal deformity is a frequent presentation. Earlier approaches to ankle replacement considered moderate and severe coronal plane deformities to be relative and, in some cases, absolute contraindications to TAR, with evidence demonstrating early failure in patients with these deformities. Wood and colleagues previously reported that edge-loading developed more commonly in patients with a pre-operative varus or valgus deformity exceeding 15° and suggested that the presence of preoperative deformity negatively influenced survivorship.[10,11] Similarly, Doets and colleagues[12] reported that preoperative coronal plane deformities were difficult to correct at the time of TAR and that it frequently resulted in "instability, subluxation of the bearing and ultimately failure". Doets suggested varus or valgus deformities greater than 10° be an "absolute" contraindication to ankle arthroplasty. In 2004, Haskell and colleagues[13] stated the coronal plane deformities were poorly understood in TAR and echoed other authors, reporting edge loading of the implant to be substantially present in cases with preoperative deformity above 10°.

Despite the initial concerns regarding coronal plane deformity in second-generation ankle implants, increasing survivorship with favorable clinical and functional outcomes led to significant improvement in prosthesis design and development of surgical techniques, with an emphasis on mitigating external forces that would jeopardize future success. Studies have supported the notion that total ankle arthroplasty is feasible for patients with preoperative severe coronal plane deformity, and that it does not significantly increase the risk of failure or postoperative complications. Hobson and colleagues[14] suggested the procedure can be performed in patients with a preoperative coronal plane deformity up to 30° without increasing the risk of failure and complications. According to Queen and colleagues,[15] TAR resulted in improved clinical and functional outcomes, even in cases where there was preoperative tibiotalar misalignment. Positive outcomes were observed if postoperative alignment was corrected to a neutral position. Lee and Lee[16] demonstrated that satisfactory outcomes can be achieved without increasing complication rates in ankles with severe coronal plane deformity and suggests that total ankle arthroplasty may be considered in cases where the deformity is greater than 20°. These studies suggest that obtaining appropriate postoperative alignment and crucial neutralization of external deforming forces of the foot and leg is a more important factor than preoperative deformity in determining the success of total ankle arthroplasty.

Varus Deformity

Patients with end-stage varus ankle arthritis present frequently and often have a subjective history of lateral ligament insufficiency and low-grade repetitive trauma. They typically report both medial and lateral ankle pain in addition to lateral column foot overload symptoms. Special attention must be given to any objective muscular imbalance and or the presence of peroneal tendon injury. The sitting examination with or without fluoroscopic examination is crucial in surgical decision making in these cases. Significant rigid deformity or inability to reduce the talus to neutral or past neutral will clue surgeons into a more complex deformity that may require significant bone work in addition to standard soft tissue balancing. In some cases, if significant extra-articular osteotomies or fusion procedures are anticipated, then a staged approach may be prudent. There is no consensus on when staging a varus deformity is necessary, but the surgeon's experience and comfort level, in addition to the morbidity of a staged procedure, should be considered for each individual case. TAR may not be suitable for all patients and in some cases the decision to pursue arthrodesis may be prudent.

In patients deemed suitable for TAR, authors have described what seem to be more universally accepted surgical techniques and algorithms for the varus deformity. In 2009, Kim and colleagues[17] compared 23 varus aligned ankles to 22 neutral aligned ankles with their novel algorithmic approach to the varus ankle deformity. They concluded that clinical improvement of the varus ankle was comparable to the neutral ankle when ancillary procedures were performed. Shock and colleagues[18] described a similar approach to the varus ankle deformity with special attention given to the necessity of reversing talar malposition into its neutral and fully reduced position. In addition to previously accepted surgical steps, there is an emphasis on the importance of addressing the lateral talofibular osseous structures with thorough debridement to allow for talar reduction. They concluded that soft tissue balancing and reestablishment of a plantigrade foot and neutral ankle resulted in successful outcomes in moderate to severe varus deformity (**Fig. 3**).

The universally accepted first step in the varus ankle is a thorough release of the deltoid ligament's deep and often superficial structures, which can be accomplished from

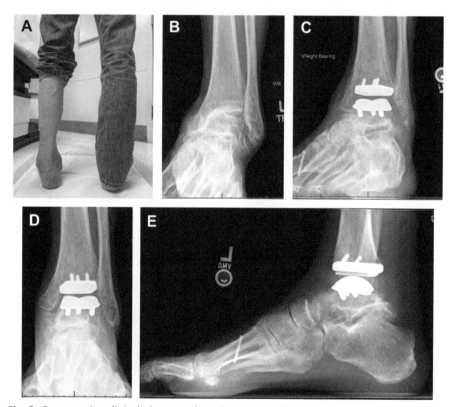

Fig. 3. Preoperative clinical photograph and mortise radiograph demonstrating end-stage ankle arthritis with varus deformity of the ankle joint secondary to chronic lateral ankle ligament laxity (*A, B*). Postoperative radiographs demonstrating full correction of ankle arthritis with varus deformity. Ancillary procedures to correct the varus deformity and balance the foot involved deltoid release, lateral gutter widening, modified Brostrum, and elevating first metatarsal osteotomy (*C–E*).

the anterior incision or a second incision as necessary. The surgeon continually assesses the ability to manually correct the talus into neutral alignment and the subsequent steps of the procedure are dependent on the ability to realign the talus to neutral. Once the deltoid ligament is addressed, it is important to evaluate any remaining medial soft tissue contracture and lateral talofibular gutter. Varus deformity often leads to significant osteophyte formation and distal fibular osseous adaption, which should be resected to achieve a neutral talar position in the mortise (**Fig. 4**). Although lateral gutter debridement can often be done through the anterior incision, a secondary incision along the lateral ankle may be necessary for better visualization and thorough removal of bone. This lateral incision is especially useful when lateral ligament plication or peroneal tendon work is needed for balancing the ankle implant. If lateral gutter debridement is complete but the talus is still not neutral, the surgeon may need to return to the medial ankle and consider further soft tissue releases, such as lengthening or releasing the posterior tibial tendon or releasing the talo-navicular joint capsule and spring ligament. In most mild to moderate varus deformities, a neutral

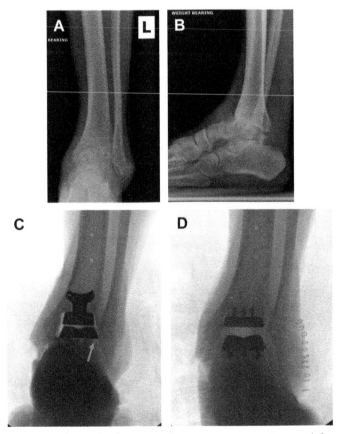

Fig. 4. Preoperative radiographs demonstrating severe congruent varus deformity of the ankle joint in a 50-year-old male with end-stage ankle arthritis (*A, B*). Intraoperative image on image intensifier demonstrating adequate varus correction after deltoid release and posterior tibial tendon lengthening. However, note the remaining medial talar translation causing offset of the talar component as indicated by red arrows (*C*). Centering of talus achieved by widening lateral gutter through saw cut of fibular malleolus (*D*).

talus can be achieved at this stage, allowing bone cutting for the ankle implant. It is crucial to align the talus to neutral so that tibial and talar bone resection cuts can be made parallel to each other, ensuring a neutral alignment of the ankle implant. In situations of severe varus where achieving talar neutralization is difficult, the surgeon may consider performing a medial malleolar osteotomy as described by Doets.[12] This requires a high level of surgical experience and skill, as the surgeon may need to fine tune tibial and talar cuts and consider further soft tissue procedures to achieve the crucial balance for the ankle implant.

After achieving neutral ankle balance and addressing any deforming soft tissue forces, bone cuts for the chosen implant can be made. It is understood that preoperative motion greatly affects range of motion in TAR surgery. Patients with limited preoperative motion are less likely to achieve higher postoperative ROM (range of motion) compared with those with more preoperative movement.[19] After choosing the appropriate polyethylene insert, ancillary lateral ligament plication may be required. Once soft tissue balancing is completed, the surgeon should evaluate any remaining foot deformity that could cause abnormal force. A lateral displacement or Dwyer osteotomy may be necessary if the calcaneus is still in a varus position. Similarly, if the medial forefoot appears plantarflexed or if there is forefoot valgus, an elevating osteotomy of the forefoot should be performed. Forefoot deformities are common in the varus ankle, and the experienced surgeon can perform this procedure with appropriate work-up and examination.

Ankle equinus deformity associated with a tight gastro-soleus complex can be present in the varus ankle and must be evaluated and diagnosed. The surgeon may address it at the beginning or mid-way through the operation, but this must be done with trials in place or after final component placement to avoid malleolar fracture.

Valgus Deformity

Valgus degenerative ankle arthritis is less common than varus deformities.[20] Although patients with valgus deformity related to previous trauma are in the minority, the overwhelming majority have pes plano valgus deformities of the foot that contribute to the valgus degeneration of the ankle. These feet can be rigid or flexible, and the multiplanar deforming forces add complexity when dealing with painful valgus ankle arthritis. When planning TAR in the valgus ankle, the key to success is the surgeon's ability to balance the implant over a plantigrade foot.[21–24] Given the complexities related to foot reconstruction and the multiprocedural approach necessary, many surgeons will choose to stage foot reconstruction and TAR into separate procedures to reduce patient risk and complications while ensuring the success of achieving a plantigrade foot prior to undertaking TAR (**Fig. 5**).

Deltoid ligament integrity is paramount, and the surgeon should have a high index of suspicion for possible deltoid ligament incompetence. Dynamic assessment under fluoroscopy can be useful but a preoperative MRI may be necessary. As with most flatfoot deformities, a high majority of these patients will demonstrate gastric-soleal equinus deformity. Like the varus ankle, surgeons should assess the ability to reduce the foot deformity. A supple foot may indicate less need for significant ancillary bone procedures, whereas a rigid deformity is likely to require rearfoot arthrodesis procedures to achieve appropriate foot balancing.

If staged surgical correction of the foot is necessary prior to TAR, the index procedure is typically performed at a minimum of 4 to 6 weeks prior to the planned joint replacement. Many authors recommend relocating the talus into neutral mortise position before foot alignment procedures and securing it with pins or intra-articular cement.[21,22] Realignment procedures should proceed from proximal to distal, with

128

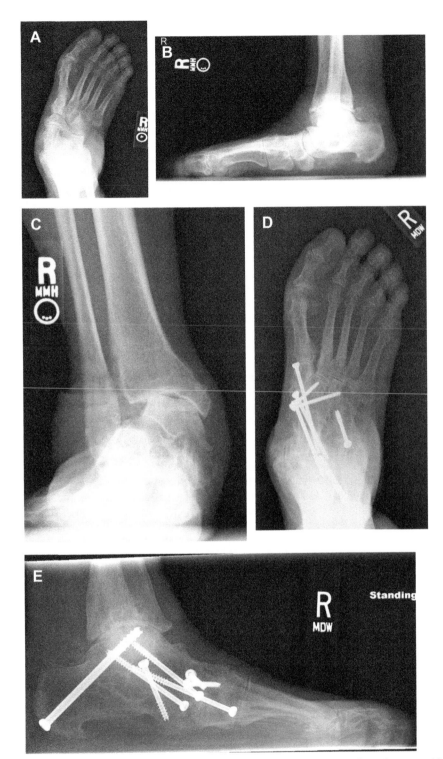

Fig. 5. Preoperative radiographs of an advanced flat foot deformity with end-stage ankle arthritis in significant valgus deformity of the joint (*A–C*). Surgical correction was staged with triple arthrodesis being the initial surgery (*D–F*). Postoperative ankle radiographs 2 years after stage 2 procedure (total ankle replacement), demonstrating satisfactory alignment of ankle with a plantigrade foot (*G, H*).

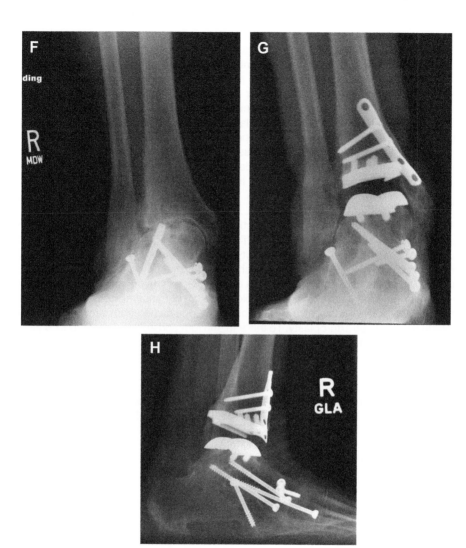

Fig. 5. (*continued*).

the goal of achieving an appropriately aligned talo-calcaneal unit and a competent medial column to neutralize any valgus thrust that would be placed upon the planned ankle prosthesis.[21] In cases of flexible pes plano valgus, corrective osteotomies and soft tissue procedures involving the posterior tibial tendon and the deltoid ligament may be necessary. In rigid deformity, arthrodesis through the subtalar, talonavicular, and often the calcaneocuboid joint may be required. If deltoid incompetence is confirmed after alignment, it should be addressed as the final step of the first-stage procedure, using the surgeon's preferred repair technique. The second-stage TAR procedure should be performed within a timeframe that minimizes patient down time but sufficient for adequate healing and successful outcome. When deltoid ligament reconstruction is undertaken, caution should be exercised in delaying the TAR, as it could compromise the initial repair due to abnormal forces resulting from remaining intra-articular valgus deformity.[21]

Achieving appropriate foot alignment in the first stage can simplify prosthesis placement in stage 2. In some cases, lateral ligament release may be necessary, along with talar body and gutter debridement to maintain neutral talar alignment. If not performed at the index procedure, a gastroc-soleal release should be considered prior to tibial and talar bone cuts. Once neutral talar position is achieved, tibial bone removal cuts can be made parallel to the mechanical axis of the tibia to correct any residual valgus adaptation at the distal tibia. Similarly, the talus can be cut parallel to the tibia and the chosen implant inserted. During polyethylene insert trialing, close attention is paid to ligament balancing. A final assessment of appropriate rearfoot and forefoot balance is performed, and any residual deformity that could adversely affect implant stability or balance can be addressed at the surgeon's discretion.

Periprosthetic Infection

Periprosthetic infection (PJI) is a devastating complication of implant arthroplasty for both the patient and the surgeon. This difficult outcome requires prolonged treatment and causes significant patient morbidity including mobility challenges, physical deconditioning, work disability, and psychological distress, while also incurring substantial financial costs. The care process can be all-consuming, and even more concerning, the infection may prove intractable. Although our understanding of PJI in TAR remains incomplete, we can draw upon the knowledge gained from similar complications in hip and knee arthroplasty. To this end, the foot and ankle workgroup's conclusions from the 2018 International Consensus Meeting on Musculoskeletal Infection form the foundation of prevention, diagnosis, and treatment of this problem.[25]

Incidence

Recent large database reviews in the United States show the prevalence of PJI in TAR to be between 1% and 4.2%.[26–28] Single institutions with a large series of patients report a range of 0.72% to 3.2% (Kaiser Permanente Northern CA, 967 patients, 2010–2018, average 7.5 year follow-up. Unpublished data).[29,30] In Kaiser Permanente Northern California, the incidence is 0.72% (Kaiser Permanente Northern CA, 967 patients, 2010–2018, average 7.5 year follow-up. Unpublished data). With the increasing adoption of TAR, the incidence of septic revision procedures has been on the rise. A recent National Inpatient Sample database study demonstrated a 256% increase in septic revision TARs between 2005 and 2017, with projections indicating a potential escalation of between 22% and 130% by 2030.[31]

Risk Factors and Prevention

The primary risk factors for PJI include the patient's immune response, the surgical environment, and the surgeon's practices. Microbes can enter the surgical site through hematogenous or exogenous routes; the latter is more common. TAR presents unique infection risks because the soft tissues are often unforgiving. The common anterior midline approach, where subcutaneous tissues are scant, demands meticulous soft tissue handling. Skin tension may increase with edema, further escalating the risk of wound complications. Patients undergoing TAR frequently have a history of trauma and previous surgeries, which may cause full-thickness scarring and impede wound healing. Most concerning, a previous soft tissue breach may provide a nidus for dormant infection that can persist for years. Therefore, a detailed patient history is essential for identifying risk factors for PJI.

Current guidelines for PJI prevention in TAR are limited, with most recommendations derived from protocols developed for hip and knee arthroplasty. The authors primarily adhere to these established conventions.

Host Factors
- Optimize nutritional status: albumin ≥ 3.5 g/dL, total lymphocyte count ≥1500 cells/mL, zinc ≥ 5 mg/dL, transferrin ≥ 200 mg/dL[32]
- Optimize glycemic control in patients with diabetes mellitus: ideally, blood glucose ≤140 mg/dL on day of surgery.[10] There is disagreement in the literature about optimal HgA1c. Our preference is ≤ 7.4%.
- BMI (body mass index) ≤30: based on hip and knee PJI, conflicting data for ankle[28,30,32]
- BMI ≥19[28]
- Stop tobacco use–conflicting data[28,30]
- Control immune-modulating comorbidities: peripheral vascular disease, chronic lung disease, hypothyroidism[28]; inflammatory bowel disease[33]; inflammatory arthritis–conflicting data[28,30]
- Careful skin assessment for wounds

Environmental factors[32,34]
- Immediately prior to procedure: surgical site hair removal with clipper, skin preparation with alcohol-containing agent
- Timely and weight-based administration of antibiotic prophylaxis
- Decrease operating room traffic
- Use iodine-impregnated drapes
- Efficient ventilation system
- Optimize surgical efficiency

Additional considerations
- Avoid TAR within 3 months of corticosteroid injection[35]
- Chlorhexidine antiseptic wipes 48 hours prior to surgery[36]
- Brief wound bath with dilute povidone-iodine solution prior to implantation[36]
- Implantation technique: no touch method, avoid implant touching skin[36]
- Minimize blood loss[36]

Definition and Diagnosis

Statistically significant parameters unique to diagnosis of PJI in TAR have not been determined because data have been limited to date. The definition for PJI in hip and knee arthroplasty was developed by the International Consensus Group on Periprosthetic Joint Infection and based on the Musculoskeletal Infection Society (MSIS).[37] Acute infections occur within 90 days of surgery, whereas chronic infections develop after 90 days. Each type of infection has different criterion thresholds. Diagnosis requires at least 1 major criterion and at least 3 of 5 minor criteria (**Table 1**). A validated diagnostic odds ratio has been established for minor criteria.[38] Most TAR literature uses the MSIS criteria to classify PJI.[30,39,40] However, some arthroplasty surgeons follow the Infectious Disease Society of America guidelines, which define acute PJI as occurring within 4 weeks of surgery or less than 3 weeks of symptoms in hematogenous presentations. Infections that manifest beyond this time frame are considered chronic.[41]

The most common pathogens in ankle PJI are *Staphylococcus aureus* and coagulase-negative staphylococci.[42] *Staphylococcus aureus* is responsible for most acute ankle PJI.[43] Its toxins are highly virulent, and the organism is capable of rapidly forming biofilm within 2 to 3 weeks of infection.[43] Coagulase-negative staphylococci, by contrast, has low-virulence but also forms dense biofilm and is responsible for most chronic ankle PJI.[42] Chronic cases may also be polymicrobial.[42]

The timing of PJI presentation has significant implications for diagnosis. Acute infections, though less common, are generally easier to recognize as they often present with wound healing problems, cellulitis, drainage, or a sinus tract.[41] A recent

Table 1
Definition of Perprosthetic join infection according to the international consensus group

PJI Present When One of the Major Criteria Exists or Three Out of Five Minor Criteria Exist

Major Criteria	Two positive periprothetic cultures with phenotypically identical organisms, *OR* A sinus tract communicating with the joint, *OR*
Minor Criteria	1. Elevated serum C-reactive protein (CRP) *AND* erythrocyte sedimentation rate (ESR) 2. Elevated synovial fluid white blood cell (WBC) count *OR* ++ change on leukocyte esterase test strip 3. Elevated synovial fluid polymorphonuclear neutrophil percentage (PMN%) 4. Positive histologial analysis of perprosthetic tissue 5. A single positive culture

The Threshold for the Minor Diagnostic Criteria

Criterion	Acute PJI (<90 d)	Chronic PJI (>90 d)
Erythrocyte sedimentation rate (mm/h)	Not helpful. No threshold was determined	30
C-reactive protein (mg/L)	100	10
Synovia white blood cell count (cells/μL)	10,000	3000
Synovial polymorphonuclear(%)	90	80
Leukocyte esterase	+ Or ++	+ Or ++
Histologic analysis of tissue	>5 neutrophils per high power field in 5 high power fields (× 400)	Same as acute

This is an adaptation of the musculoskeletal infection society definition of PJI.

From Parvizi J, Gehrke T. Definition of periprosthetic joint infection. J Arthroplasty 2014;29(7):1331.

systematic review found the rate of acute PJI in TAR to be only 8.8% with the first 3 months.[26] In contrast, chronic PJI is more common in TAR and can be subtle and challenging to detect. Clinical suspicion is paramount, and while component loosening is strongly suggestive of PJI in the hip and knee, aseptic loosening is more common in the ankle. Persistent pain without other clear causes is a compelling symptom for PJI. In cases where the diagnosis is uncertain, the combination of a positive alpha defensin and synovial C-reactive protein above 3 is highly reliable for diagnosis.[38]

Pathogen identification is critical to guide treatment in PJI but can be difficult in the chronic presentation. Between 3 and 6 intraoperative tissue samples should be sent for culture and incubated for 5 to 14 days.[44,45] Both implant sonication and prolonged culture incubation show promise to improve culture yield. In culture-negative cases, molecular methods such as next-generation sequencing (NGS) have been shown to rapidly identify pathogens in both synovial fluid and tissue samples.[46,47] Although NGS is not readily available in most health care systems, it may eventually transform the existing tedious and intensive diagnostic process in the clinical microbiology laboratory.[48]

Treatment

Beyond the challenges of diagnosis and pathogen identification, it can be difficult for the TAR surgeon to assist the patient in making an informed decision regarding the successful treatment of ankle PJI. Patients must be educated about the risks of failure, and the surgeon must also ascertain their own risk tolerance.

Single-stage treatment with debridement, antibiotics, and implant retention (DAIR) is common in the management of acute PJI. This approach is inherently appealing because of the morbidity of 2-stage treatment, but it requires meticulous technique. The success rate for single-stage PJI treatment in hip and knee arthroplasty for patients who meet specific criteria approaches 90%.[49]

Unfortunately, this outcome has not been attained in TAR. Treatment of acute ankle PJI can be very challenging, particularly in the setting of soft tissue compromise, which is not uncommon[50] (**Fig. 6**). Two recent large patient series demonstrated a

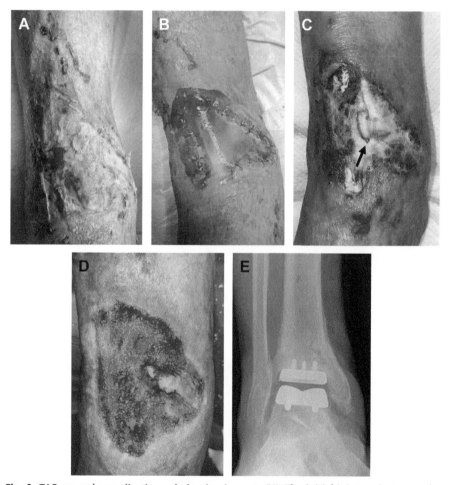

Fig. 6. TAR wound complication culminating in acute PJI. The initial joint aspirate was dry. (*A*) Early on the tendon sheath and joint capsule was intact. (*B*) The culture-negative wound was debrided and covered with a bilayer matrix wound dressing. (*C*) The wound quickly deteriorated and tracked deep to the joint within 2 weeks (tendon excised, exposed tibial component in center of wound–*black arrow*). (*D*) Within 4 weeks of the index procedure the patient was treated with irrigation, debridement, and polyethylene exchange with twice weekly washout for 4 weeks until cultures were negative and the deeper tissue layers healed. The components were not loose. The remainder of the wound healed over 3 months as inflammatory markers normalized. (*E*) Radiograph at 8 months. The patient was functioning well with no ankle pain and normal inflammatory markers. The patient is on life-long antibiotic suppression owing to the risk of residual pathogens.

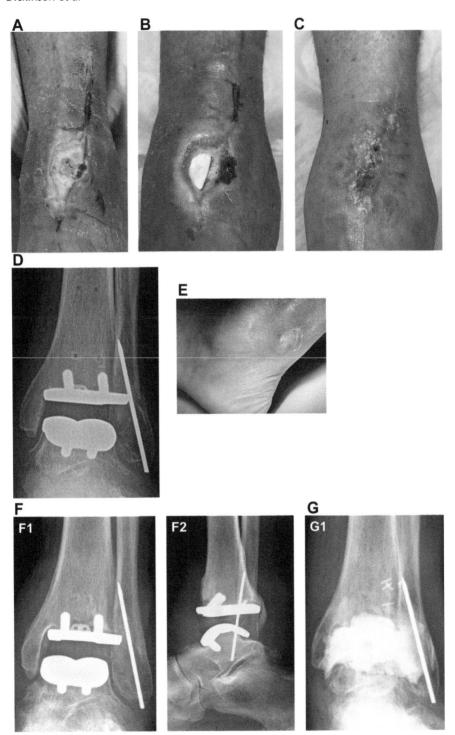

Fig. 7. TAR wound complication followed by chronic PJI. Serial joint aspirations during the first few postoperative weeks were culture negative with synovial white blood cell (WBC) count well below infection threshold. Inflammatory markers were not significantly elevated. (*A*) Wound at 2.5 weeks and (*B*) 3.5 weeks. Joint capsule intact. (*C*) Wound debridement

G   **H**

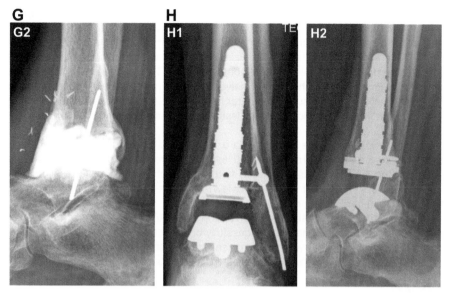

Fig. 7. (*continued*).

40% to 54% long-term failure rate for single-stage treatment of acute PJI.[29,42] Indeed, there is disagreement about the optimal approach to treatment of acute PJI in TAR. In one of these series, the surgeons who prefer DAIR believed "the ~50/50 odds of success are worth the risk if a staged revision with antibiotic cement spacer can be avoided. Those who prefer the more aggressive approach cite the 54% failure rate as support for going straight to staged treatment".[29]

Early formation of biofilm around the ankle prosthesis, including the bone-implant interface, may complicate distinguishing acute from chronic infection in some cases. In fact, some acute hematogenous PJI may be low-grade chronic infection, similar to indolent osteomyelitis, resulting from early contamination. This highlights the need for more aggressive treatment strategies.

Most cases of TAR PJI are chronic, which is similar to entrenched osteomyelitis. A staged treatment approach is essential: meticulous debridement and irrigation (often guided by methylene-blue injection), explantation, insertion of polymethylmethacrylate

---

with tendon excision and application of bilayer matrix dressing, healed within 6 weeks. (*D*) Radiograph at 4 months. Patient had no pain and normal inflammatory markers. (*E*) Twenty months later, following dental procedures and treatment of gluteal abscess and while traveling overseas, the patient presented with a painful, warm, swollen ankle, and a draining sinus. Synovial WBC count 7000 significantly elevated inflammatory markers. (*F*) Radiographs depict osteolysis. (F1,F2) AP and lateral radiographs depicting osteolysis of the tibial tray. (*G*) (G1,G2) AP and lateral radiographs after treatment with explantation, methylene-blue driven debridement and irrigation, placement of PMMA antibiotic spacer, and 6 weeks of IV antibiotics for *Staphylococcus epidermidis* infection. (*H*) (H1,H2) AP and Lateral radiographsat 3 years following reiplantation with stemmed components (assistance from Jack Schuberth, DPM): performed at 3 months when serial inflammatory markers were normal for a month and aspiration of cement block culture negative with low WBC. A minor superficial incisional wound developed but healed quickly. The patient has been functional without pain since.

antibiotic-impregnated spacer, culture-directed intravenous antibiotics, and repeat debridement/irrigation as necessary (**Fig. 7**). Once the wound has healed, the patient may load the cement spacer with brace support.[51] Reimplantation should occur only once inflammatory markers have normalized and fluid aspiration about the block demonstrates no pathogens, often several months or more. Tissue samples should be obtained for microbiology and histologic analysis during reimplantation. Although revision implant systems afford the surgeon greater flexibility for successful reconstruction, the impaired soft tissue envelope is no less forgiving and wound healing can be problematic.

Two-stage revision is the gold standard for chronic PJI in hip and knee implant arthroplasty with success rates over 90%.[41,51] Two recent large TAR series have demonstrated similar results for staged treatment of chronic PJI, with a failure rate of 9% to 10%.[42,52] Another systemic review and meta-analysis have demonstrated no failures for 1- or 2-stage revision in TAR PJI.[53]

In some cases, reimplantation is not an option after TAR explantation for PJI. In such situations, some patients may be successfully converted to arthrodesis,[42,50,54] whereas others may be treated with a permanent cement spacer.[51] Unfortunately, some patients never clear their infection and require amputation.[53]

SUMMARY

TAR with modern implant systems has demonstrated promising outcomes for patients with end-stage ankle arthritis. Consistent success and reproducibility, particularly for arthritis with challenging deformities, requires thorough evaluation and careful patient selection, systematic implementation of ancillary procedures, staged surgery as indicated, and precise balancing of the prosthesis on a plantigrade foot. Patient risk stratification, meticulous tissue handling, technical efficiency, and methodical infection control measures are required to minimize the risk for a devastating prosthetic joint infection.

CLINICS CARE POINTS

- A deltoid ligament release is typically a necessary step for the correction of a varus deformity.
- Whether or not a 2-stage surgery is required, a plantigrade foot is critical to obtain optimum balancing and stability of the prosthesis.
- The treatment of ankle prosthetic joint infections requires an aggressive approach of multiple surgical debridements and long-term antibiotics. The decision between DAIR and explantation with later reimplantation is at the discretion of the surgeon based on the clinical scenario, but implant retention is at the risk of an approximately 50% failure rate.

DISCLOSURES

The authors have nothing to disclose.

REFERENCES

1. Glazebrook M, Daniels T, Younger A, et al. Comparison of health-related quality of life between patients with end-stage ankle and hip arthrosis. J Bone Joint Surg Am 2008;90(3):499–505.

2. Saltzman CL, Zimmerman MB, O'Rourke M, et al. Impact of comorbidities on the measurement of health in patients with ankle osteoarthritis. J Bone Joint Surg Am 2006;88(11):2366–72.

3. Coester LM, Saltzman CL, Leupold J, et al. Long-term results following ankle arthrodesis for post-traumatic arthritis. J Bone Joint Surg Am 2001;83(2):219–28.

4. Espinosa N, Walti M, Favre P, et al. Misalignment of total ankle components can induce high joint contact pressures. J Bone Joint Surg Am 2010;92(5):1179–87.

5. Morgan EF, Unnikrisnan GU, Hussein AI. Bone mechanical properties in healthy and diseased States. Annu Rev Biomed Eng 2018;20:119–43.

6. Nielsen NM, Saito GH, Sanders AE, et al. Sagittal tibiotalar alignment may not affect functional outcomes in fixed-bearing total ankle replacement: a retrospective cohort study. HSS J 2020;16(Suppl 2):300–4.

7. Najefi AA, Ghani Y, Goldberg A. Role of rotation in total ankle replacement. Foot Ankle Int 2019;40(12):1358–67.

8. McKearney DA, Stender CJ, Cook BK, et al. Altered range of motion and plantar pressure in anterior and posterior malaligned total ankle arthroplasty: a cadaveric gait study. J Bone Joint Surg Am 2019;101(18):e93.

9. Le V, Escudero M, Symes M, et al. Impact of sagittal talar inclination on total ankle replacement failure. Foot Ankle Int 2019;40(8):900–4.

10. Wood PL, Deakin S. Total ankle replacement. The results in 200 ankles. J Bone Joint Surg Br 2003;85(3):334–41.

11. Wood PL, Prem H, Sutton C. Total ankle replacement: medium-term results in 200 Scandinavian total ankle replacements. J Bone Joint Surg Br 2008;90(5):605–9.

12. Doets HC, Brand R, Nelissen RG. Total ankle arthroplasty in inflammatory joint disease with use of two mobile-bearing designs [published correction appears in J Bone Joint Surg Am. 2007 Jan;89(1):158]. J Bone Joint Surg Am 2006; 88(6):1272–84.

13. Haskell A, Mann RA. Ankle arthroplasty with preoperative coronal plane deformity: short-term results. Clin Orthop Relat Res 2004;424:98–103.

14. Hobson SA, Karantana A, Dhar S. Total ankle replacement in patients with significant pre-operative deformity of the hindfoot. J Bone Joint Surg Br 2009;91(4): 481–6.

15. Queen RM, Adams SB Jr, Viens NA, et al. Differences in outcomes following total ankle replacement in patients with neutral alignment compared with tibiotalar joint malalignment. J Bone Joint Surg Am 2013;95(21):1927–34.

16. Lee GW, Lee KB. Outcomes of total ankle arthroplasty in ankles with >20° of coronal plane deformity. J Bone Joint Surg Am 2019;101(24):2203–11.

17. Kim BS, Choi WJ, Kim YS, et al. Total ankle replacement in moderate to severe varus deformity of the ankle. J Bone Joint Surg Br 2009;91(9):1183–90.

18. Shock RP, Christensen JC, Schuberth JM. Total ankle replacement in the varus ankle. J Foot Ankle Surg 2011;50(1):5–10.

19. Ajis A, Henriquez H, Myerson M. Postoperative range of motion trends following total ankle arthroplasty. Foot Ankle Int 2013;34(5):645–56.

20. Horisberger M, Valderrabano V, Hintermann B. Posttraumatic ankle osteoarthritis after ankle-related fractures. J Orthop Trauma 2009;23(1):60–7.

21. Schuberth JM, Christensen JC, Seidenstricker CL. Total ankle replacement with severe valgus deformity: technique and surgical strategy. J Foot Ankle Surg 2017;56(3):618–27.

22. Cottom JM, DeVries JG, Hyer CF, et al. Current techniques in total ankle arthroplasty. Clin Podiatr Med Surg 2022;39(2):273–93.

23. Demetracopoulos CA, Cody EA, Adams SB Jr, et al. Outcomes of total ankle arthroplasty in moderate and severe valgus deformity. Foot Ankle Spec 2019;12(3): 238–45.

24. Halai MM, Pinsker E, Mann MA, et al. Should 15° of valgus coronal-plane deformity be the upper limit for a total ankle arthroplasty? Bone Joint Lett J 2020; 102-B(12):1689–96.

25. Aiyer A, Raikin S, Parvizi J. 2018 International consensus meeting on musculoskeletal infection: findings of the foot and ankle work Group. Foot Ankle Int 2019;40(1_suppl):1S.

26. Miner SA, Martucci JA, Brigido SA, et al. Time to revision after periprosthetic joint infection in total ankle arthroplasty: a systematic review. J Foot Ankle Surg 2023; 62(1):186–90.

27. McKenna BJ, Cook J, Cook EA, et al. Total ankle arthroplasty survivorship: a meta-analysis. J Foot Ankle Surg 2020;59(5):1040–8.

28. Althoff A, Cancienne JM, Cooper MT, et al. Patient-related risk factors for periprosthetic ankle joint infection: an analysis of 6977 total ankle arthroplasties. J Foot Ankle Surg 2018;57(2):269–72.

29. Lachman JR, Ramos JA, DeOrio JK, et al. Outcomes of acute hematogenous periprosthetic joint infection in total ankle arthroplasty treated with irrigation, debridement, and polyethylene exchange. Foot Ankle Int 2018;39(11):1266–71.

30. Patton D, Kiewiet N, Brage M. Infected total ankle arthroplasty: risk factors and treatment options. Foot Ankle Int 2015;36(6):626–34.

31. Shah JA, Schwartz AM, Farley KX, et al. Projections and epidemiology of total ankle and revision total ankle arthroplasty in the United States to 2030 [published online ahead of print, 2022 jul 14]. Foot Ankle Spec 2022. https://doi.org/10.1177/ 19386400221109420. 19386400221109420.

32. Emara K, Hirose CB, Rogero R. What preoperative optimization should Be implemented to reduce the risk of surgical site infection/periprosthetic joint infection (SSI/PJI) in patients undergoing total ankle arthroplasty (TAA)? Foot Ankle Int 2019;40(1_suppl):6S–8S.

33. Chisari E, D'Mello D, Sherman MB, et al. Inflammatory bowel diseases increase the risk of periprosthetic joint infection. J Bone Joint Surg Am 2022;104(2):160–5.

34. Matar WY, Jafari SM, Restrepo C, et al. Preventing infection in total joint arthroplasty. J Bone Joint Surg Am 2010;92(Suppl 2):36–46.

35. Uçkay I, Hirose CB, Assal M. Does intra-articular injection of the ankle with corticosteroids increase the risk of subsequent periprosthetic joint infection (PJI) following total ankle arthroplasty (TAA)? If so, how long after a prior intra-articular injection can TAA Be safely performed? Foot Ankle Int 2019; 40(1_suppl):3S–4S.

36. Parvizi J. Periprosthetic joint infection prevention. Symposium Q: Periprosthetic joint infections of the knee: everything you need to know in 90 minutes. American Academy of Orthopaedic Surgeons Annual Meeting, March 7, 2023, Las Vegas, NV.

37. Fillingham YA, Della Valle CJ, Suleiman LI, et al. Definition of successful infection management and guidelines for reporting of outcomes after surgical treatment of periprosthetic joint infection: from the workgroup of the musculoskeletal infection society (MSIS). J Bone Joint Surg Am 2019;101(14):e69.

38. Parvizi J, Tan TL, Goswami K, et al. The 2018 definition of periprosthetic hip and knee infection: an evidence-based and validated criteria. J Arthroplasty 2018; 33(5):1309–14.e2.

39. Aynardi MC, Plöger MM, Walley KC, et al. What is the definition of acute and chronic periprosthetic joint infection (PJI) of total ankle arthroplasty (TAA)? Foot Ankle Int 2019;40(1_suppl):19S–21S.
40. Alrashidi Y, Galhoum AE, Wiewiorski M, et al. How to diagnose and treat infection in total ankle arthroplasty. Foot Ankle Clin 2017;22(2):405–23.
41. Osmon DR, Berbari EF, Berendt AR, et al. Diagnosis and management of prosthetic joint infection: clinical practice guidelines by the Infectious Diseases Society of America. Clin Infect Dis 2013;56(1):e1–25.
42. Pfahl K, Röser A, Gottschalk O, et al. Common bacteria and treatment options for the acute and chronic infection of the total ankle arthroplasty. Foot Ankle Surg 2022;28(7):1008–13.
43. Nishitani K, Sutipornpalangkul W, de Mesy Bentley KL, et al. Quantifying the natural history of biofilm formation in vivo during the establishment of chronic implant-associated Staphylococcus aureus osteomyelitis in mice to identify critical pathogen and host factors. J Orthop Res 2015;33(9):1311–9.
44. Mikkelsen DB, Pedersen C, Højbjerg T, et al. Culture of multiple peroperative biopsies and diagnosis of infected knee arthroplasties. APMIS 2006;114(6):449–52.
45. Schäfer P, Fink B, Sandow D, et al. Prolonged bacterial culture to identify late periprosthetic joint infection: a promising strategy. Clin Infect Dis 2008;47(11):1403–9.
46. Tarabichi M, Shohat N, Goswami K, et al. Diagnosis of periprosthetic joint infection: the potential of next-generation sequencing. J Bone Joint Surg Am 2018;100(2):147–54.
47. Tarabichi M, Shohat N, Goswami K, et al. Can next generation sequencing play a role in detecting pathogens in synovial fluid? Bone Joint Lett J 2018;100-B(2):127–33.
48. Goswami K, Parvizi J, Maxwell Courtney P. Current recommendations for the diagnosis of acute and chronic PJI for hip and knee-cell counts, alpha-defensin, leukocyte esterase, next-generation sequencing. Curr Rev Musculoskelet Med 2018;11(3):428–38.
49. Tschudin-Sutter S, Frei R, Dangel M, et al. Validation of a treatment algorithm for orthopaedic implant-related infections with device-retention-results from a prospective observational cohort study. Clin Microbiol Infect 2016;22(5):457.e1–4579.
50. Kessler B, Knupp M, Graber P, et al. The treatment and outcome of periprosthetic infection of the ankle: a single cohort-centre experience of 34 cases. Bone Joint Lett J 2014;96-B(6):772–7.
51. Ferrao P, Myerson MS, Schuberth JM, et al. Cement spacer as definitive management for postoperative ankle infection. Foot Ankle Int 2012;33(3):173–8.
52. Kunutsor SK, Whitehouse MR, Lenguerrand E, et al, INFORM Team. Re-infection outcomes following one- and two-stage surgical revision of infected knee prosthesis: a systematic review and meta-analysis. PLoS One 2016;11(3):e0151537.
53. Kunutsor SK, Barrett MC, Whitehouse MR, et al. Clinical effectiveness of treatment strategies for prosthetic joint infection following total ankle replacement: a systematic review and meta-analysis. J Foot Ankle Surg 2020;59(2):367–72.
54. Carlsson AS, Montgomery F, Besjakov J. Arthrodesis of the ankle secondary to replacement. Foot Ankle Int 1998;19(4):240–5.

Considerations in Charcot Reconstruction

Luke J. McCann, DPM, PT[a],*, Joseph D. Dickinson, DPM[b]

KEYWORDS

- Charcot • Reconstruction • Surgery • Diabetes • Amputation • Limb salvage

KEY POINTS

- Charcot deformity is difficult to control, leading to high rates of ulceration, infection, limb amputation.
- Aggressive stabilization is needed to prevent limb loss and preserve function.
- Timing of surgery and fixation approaches should be determined on a case-to-case basis.

INTRODUCTION

Charcot neuroarthropathy is a devastating condition that can be challenging to treat. In the best of circumstances, it is detected early and managed conservatively with nonoperative intervention, preventing loss of a plantigrade foot and future ulceration. Even in instances of early detection and aggressive nonoperative management, patients often will develop foot deformity, leading to ulceration, infection, and loss of limb or life. The two primary interventions to manage Charcot are nonoperative immobilization and surgical intervention–both with the goals of maintaining a plantigrade foot. The treatment of the former is typically achieved through casting followed by lifelong offloading and bracing. The latter approach is to alleviate bony prominences and provide a plantigrade foot to prevent future ulceration. In more severe instances where deformity and instability occur, surgical reconstruction is considered. There are various surgical techniques that can be used to reconstruct these deformities. These usually include external fixation, internal fixation, or a combination of internal and external fixation.[1] These can range from open reduction and internal fixation (ORIF) using plates and screws, intramedullary nails, and static and dynamic external fixation frames. However, there is not a strong consensus as to what the best form of treatment is for this condition. There is an overall lack of consensus regarding how to best treat these patients. Points of contention are whether to do surgery at all, and if surgery is performed, what is the optimal type of fixation used. The authors would argue that

---

[a] Kaiser South San Francisco Medical Center, 1200 El Camino Real, South San Francisco, CA 94108, USA; [b] Kaiser Oakland Medical Center, 3600 Broadway, Oakland, CA 94611, USA
* Corresponding author.
E-mail address: Luke.j.mccann@kp.org

no two cases are alike, and each should be treated in an individualized manner taking all data points into consideration. Factors such as presence of ulcer, active soft tissue or bone infection, active or quiescent Charcot process, hemoglobin A1c and diabetes control, blood flow, severity of deformity, and patient goals are all elements that influence treatment.

There are multiple studies that show the 5-year mortality can range from above 40% to 56% in patients after proximal limb amputation.[2–5] Armstrong and colleagues found that patients with a diagnosis of Charcot had a 5-year mortality of 29%.[5] A large retrospective study (n = 911) by Sohn and colleagues found patients with a Charcot diagnosis have a 7 times higher risk for amputation. They further found that Charcot in conjunction with an ulcer increased risk of amputation 12 times.[6] With high mortality rates after limb amputation, it imperative that foot and ankle surgeons do whatever possible to prevent limb loss. For this reason, many choose the path of surgical reconstruction.

One of the first considerations regarding Charcot is early detection. At Kaiser Permanente Northern California (KPNC), the authors are fortunate that their system is a close network of physicians who work together and can consult one another easily. Frequently, these patients will present with a hot red swollen foot, appearing cellulitic in nature as a possible infection.[7] Often these patients are treated first for cellulitis or gout and given additional workup for deep vein thrombosis or venous stasis. Fortunately, these patients are typically referred to the Podiatry Clinic, where Charcot is quickly ruled in or out. Because the emergency department and primary care colleagues are usually the first providers to encounter these patients, the authors feel it is important to reiterate that having a low threshold to refer to podiatry is critical. Initial recommendations would be to keep the patient nonweight-bearing if possible, obtain baseline radiographs, baseline laboratory tests, and if cellulitis is suspected, then treat the cellulitis.

Charcot is most often associated diabetic neuropathy.[7–9] Podiatrists tend to encounter Charcot more frequently.[7–9] The classic patient is one with profound neuropathy and diabetes, who develops a hot red swollen foot without necessarily having any memorable traumatic event to justify such symptoms. However, Charcot neuroarthropathy can arise in anyone with neuropathy. Although it is less common, it can be seen in neuropathy caused by excessive alcohol use, syphilis, spinal cord injuries, tabes dorsalis, leprosy/Hansen disease, and syringomyelia.[10] Charcot-inducing events can range from trauma, repetitive microtrauma, surgery, thermal injury, or drugs/medication.[10] Many times, there is not an open wound, nor is there any obvious deformity when clinically looking at the foot. Through laboratory tests, radiographs, and clinical examination, a diagnosis of Charcot can usually be made. Initial frontline treatment involves nonweight bearing total contact casting to offload, prevent progression of deformity, and allow the process to become quiescent and the deformity to consolidate. Unfortunately, in many instances, patients may end up developing a need for surgical intervention. When this occurs, there are many components to take into consideration. The authors use several basic principles to help guide the decision-making process with the understanding that no two cases are identical.

PREOPERATIVE CONSIDERATIONS
Timing of Surgery

As is often the case with Charcot, deformity occurs despite best efforts at conservative management. When cast immobilization fails, and patients develop instability, ulceration, or bony deformity, surgery is then typically considered. Without definitive literature guiding, the timing of surgery can be somewhat of an art. In the absence of bony prominence or ulceration, time is on one's side to allow the process to coalesce and consolidate prior to surgical reconstruction. It is preferable to carry out a reconstructive type of procedure once the Charcot process has become quiescent and consolidated. When this is the case, there is more stable bone stock for fixation to be placed. However, in some cases, waiting for consolidation is not an option, as deformity or ulceration ensues, creating a more pressing need for surgical management.

When deformities are mild and there is simply prominent bone on the plantar foot, one can consider an exostectomy procedure to prevent ulceration or facilitate wound closure. However, it has been the authors' experience that in many instances exostectomy can result in a chasing the bump scenario, where one ends up repeating procedures, as transfer lesions often occur. There is also the concern that removing additional bone can further destabilize the foot. When deformities are more severe and accompanied by instability, it is necessary to reduce the malalignment and stabilize the foot and ankle while the Charcot process coalesces. From a surgical standpoint, this can be carried out in a variety of ways. This article will focus on surgical management and considerations with some of the different but commonly encountered scenarios pertaining to reconstruction of the foot.

Glucose Control

An elevated hemoglobin A1c value is common with Charcot patients.[11] This puts surgeons in a bit of a conundrum, as poor glucose control raises risks of complication and infection.[12] One consideration is to perform less invasive stabilization procedures by means of percutaneous pinning, external fixation, or a combination of the two. This can be done preliminarily to stabilize the deformity while the patient works on improving glucose control as the Charcot process becomes quiescent. Once glucose control is optimized, then a more definitive correction can be performed. Every attempt to get A1c value below 8.0% should be made before definitive fixation to avoid risk of complication.[12]

Location of Charcot

Location of Charcot impacts surgical decision making. Overall, the authors find it more difficult to correct and control Charcot of the ankle and rearfoot (talonavicular joint, subtalar joint, calcaneal cuboid joint, ankle joint). This is attributed to the axial load proximally, which creates deformity in the coronal plane (**Fig. 1**). The authors published a study where they found reconstruction at the ankle or subtalar joint (STJ) carried a 3.3 times higher risk of limb amputation compared with reconstruction at the medial column.[13] The authors have found that Charcot events at the midfoot have overall better prognosis, because the deforming forces in the sagittal plane have less of an axial load, and the deforming forces can more easily be minimized. Charcot within the hindfoot and ankle should be held in a strict nonweight-bearing total contact cast (TCC) with serial radiographs and lower threshold for applying external fixation to hold out to length and prevent deformity.

Presence of Ulcer or Bone

Presence of ulceration, exposed bone, or osteomyelitis introduces additional variables that muddy the water in the surgical decision-making process. On one hand, reduction of deformity is imperative to alleviate skin tenting and allow for bony coverage and wound healing. However, careful consideration needs to be taken regarding fixation in a limb with an ulcer and/or bone involved. An existing ulcer may limit hardware placement or compromise stability. Infection should first be treated in instances where an ulcer extends close to bone or has osteomyelitis. With this scenario, it would be

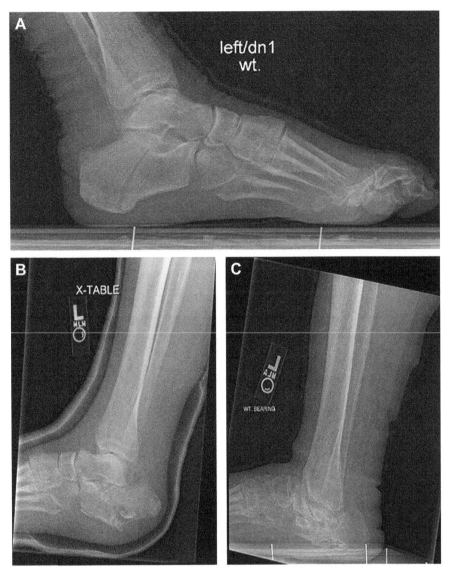

Fig. 1. Continued bone destruction and lose despite being nonweight bearing in a total contact cast (TCC).

recommended to remove any necrotic tissue or exposed bone, take bone biopsies, and attempt to achieve wound closure. The authors will frequently use antibiotic beads in addition to a long-term course of intravenous (IV) antibiotics. Their infectious disease colleagues are also consulted and become part of the team to help guide the decision-making process for antibiotic usage and need for hardware removal. Serial C-reactive protein (CRP) and erythrocyte sedimentation rate (ESR) inflammatory markers are followed to ensure down trending and resolution of infection before definitive fixation and placement of any internal hardware. Imaging studies such as MRI or WBC tagged bone scans could also be used to help guide timing. However, the authors find their use to be more beneficial in the initial diagnosis of osteomyelitis.

Additionally, one can perform serial bone biopsy before proceeding with definitive fixation; however, in their practice the authors typically rely on inflammatory markers and soft tissue healing.

SURGICAL CONSIDERATIONS
Exostectomy

Exostectomy is one of the simplest ways to address a bony prominence brought on by Charcot. This involves a straightforward incision with resection of the prominent bone. In cases where deformity is small, this can first be done to help maintain a plantigrade foot and prevent or alleviate impending ulceration. When there is exposed bone, this approach also allows for removal of possible osteomyelitis, pathologic evaluation, and possible wound closure. Bone resection is typically followed by casting/bracing to ensure adequate corrective positioning while the process coalesces. This is often more successful in consolidated deformities with focal prominence. Concerns with this approach are reactivation of the Charcot process and development of additional transfer lesions requiring additional procedures. Furthermore, resection of bone can destabilize the bony architecture causing deformity progression.

Achilles Lengthening

An Achilles tendon lengthening is recommended in all patients with a Charcot event at some point. If Charcot is detected before there is any major deformity, a percutaneous tendon Achilles lengthening (TAL) can be performed under local anesthesia, often in a clinic procedure room. Alternatively, if there is deformity requiring reduction and correction in the operating room, the Achilles tendon lengthening can be done at that time. Whether it is done initially or at time of reconstruction, the authors feel it is important to negate this deforming force.

Stabilization of Columns

Midfoot
One can divide the architecture of the foot into 3 columns and focus on fixating each to make for a stable foot. The medial column would include the first ray; the central column would include the second and third rays, and the lateral column would include the fourth and fifth rays. When using internal fixation, much attention goes to stabilizing the medial and lateral column. The authors also pay close attention to the central column, as they have frequently observed lateral and intermediate cuneiform collapse causing plantar lateral prominence. The general approach is to add robust fixation at the medial and lateral columns, where screws originating from each of these columns are used to capture and stabilize central column. This is thought of as more of a ladder approach. They have found the application of the superconstruct to be critical in maintaining correction (**Fig. 2**). This is where robust fixation is placed beyond the zone of deformity to provide added stability. With Charcot of the midfoot it would entail stabilizing distally along the metatarsals and proximally into the rearfoot. Medial column stabilization would include fixation from distal first metatarsal into the talus. Lateral stabilization would entail fixation across the calcaneal cuboid joint. Additionally, the authors typically prefer to stabilize at the subtalar joint also, which creates a more rigid pyramid structure.

Ankle/rearfoot
Axial loading and coronal plane deformity is of concern with Charcot at this level. The basic concept here would be to achieve a rearfoot with the talus stacked on the calcaneus, which sits in the ankle mortise directly below the tibia. The primary goal here is to

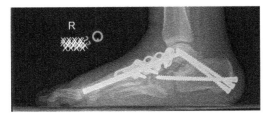

Fig. 2. Pyramid construct seen from a lateral radiograph.

keep the rearfoot in line with tibia in order to restore mechanical axis of the lower leg. With axial load forces being so powerful, the authors usually find this is best achieved with a combination of internal and external fixation (**Figs. 3–5**).

Minimally Invasive Versus Open Reduction

When deciding on a definitive fixation approach, there are several factors to consider that may sway one towards a minimally invasive approach versus open reduction approach. A minimally invasive approach should be favored in situations where there is concern for soft tissue healing or soft existing tissue compromise. Chronic edema, inelastic and contracted soft tissue, poor vascularity, or questionable ability to heal a larger incision are reasons to consider a minimally invasive approach. A minimally invasive approach should also be considered for patients with end-stage renal disease. A specific example would be a patient with severe abducto-valgus deformity that is then brought into rectus alignment. In this case, the lateral soft tissue may be contracted and not able to tolerate wound closure in addition to a large incision with bulky hardware. This potentially would create a risk for dehiscence and tissue compromise. In this scenario, a minimally invasive approach via beaming or beaming combined with external fixation may be a better option. A healthy balance between robust stabilization and minimizing soft tissue compromise must be achieved. Generally, the authors feel there is more of a role for minimally invasive surgery in consolidated deformities where the soft tissue has adapted. Otherwise, the authors feel

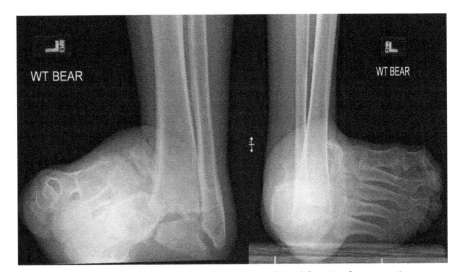

Fig. 3. Example of coronal plane deformity using combined fixation for correction.

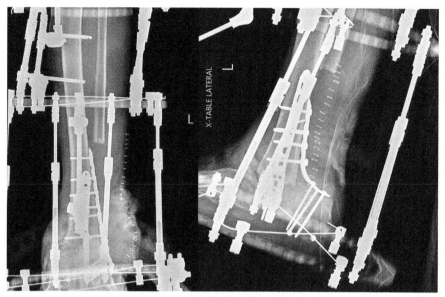

Fig. 4. Placement of internal and external fixation.

that if the soft tissue is likely able to tolerate a larger open incision approach, then an open incision approach should be pursued.

External Fixation

In instances of acute Charcot, basic stabilization is important while the destructive phase transitions into the reparative and coalesced phases. Early in the Charcot process, it is often not feasible to perform a more involved open reconstruction with multiple incisions and implanted hardware in the presence of fragmented bone and poorly

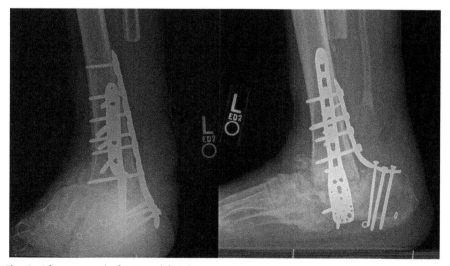

Fig. 5. After removal of external fixation.

controlled diabetes. When there is soft tissue compromise, an active soft tissue or bone infection, or when the blood glucose/HgbA1c is grossly uncontrolled, external fixation should be considered. Stabilization can be achieved with percutaneous fixation and stabilization using external fixation. This allows for adequate deformity reduction while maintaining the soft tissue envelope and avoiding large incision portals. The authors' choice typically involves percutaneous pinning followed by placement of an Ilizarov type ring fixation as opposed to use of a delta frame. The authors feel ring fixators provide more points of stability and better distribute forces.

Internal Fixation

At the midfoot, the authors favor an approach that beams the medial column with intramedullary fixation in combination with a medial caterpillar type plate. With the addition of plating, it allows for driving screws across the central column to create additional rebar for added stability. Fixation would typically entail an intramedullary beam at the first ray from the metatarsal head into the talus in conjunction with a robust plate (**Fig. 6**). The screws from the medial plate are driven across the central column stabilizing the cuneiforms and central metatarsals. The lateral column can then be plated also with screws being driven from lateral column medially to capture the talus and navicular. Alternatively, one can drive an intramedullary nail along the lateral column. However, the authors have frequently seen the lateral column nail break or migrate, necessitating removal. From a procedural standpoint, a typical scenario would follow like this: reduce, prepare the joints, and apply temporary plate fixation to the medial column first using k-wire. Next an intramedullary beam would be driven from head of the first metatarsal to the talus. The medial plate would then be fixated with screws stabilizing the medial and central columns. Finally, the lateral column fixation would be achieved with a combination of plate and screws, again with screws purchasing both the lateral column and the central column (**Fig. 7**).

At the rearfoot and ankle, the authors will almost always combine internal and external fixation. Usually with arthrodesis involving any combination of the talonavicular joint, subtalar joint, and ankle joint, the authors will place rigid internal hardware followed by an external ring fixator. It is felt that addition of an external fixator better

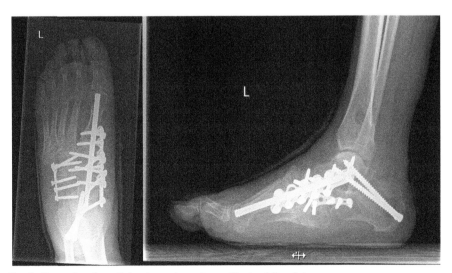

Fig. 6. Example of medial column beaming with straddle plate.

protects against axial load deforming forces and will protect the internal hardware. There are various techniques deployed to achieve this, which are determined on a case-by-case basis. The authors tend to favor dual plating and/or consideration for use of intramedullary tibial-talo-calcaneal fixation. In instances with bone loss where the ankle joint is being fused, the fibula can be used for bone grafting purposes. The external fixator remains in place between 10 to 12 weeks.

POSTOPERATIVE CONSIDERATIONS
Timing to Weight Bearing

For post-reconstruction success, it is imperative that weight-bearing restrictions are followed. The authors post-surgical reconstruction periods of nonweight bearing typically range from 8 to 12 weeks at a minimum. With external fixation, it is a 12-week period of nonweight bearing in the frame. Because the Charcot process can take anywhere from several weeks to several months to become quiescent, there will be times where a longer duration of nonweight bearing or minimal weight bearing will be required. Time to weight bearing should be guided by serial radiographs with evidence of bone and soft tissue healing followed by a gradual progression of weight bearing with close follow-up. A common timing sequence for patients after reconstruction would be

- Start minimal protected weight bearing in a CAM (controlled ankle motion) boot around 8 to 12 weeks once skin is healed and there is radiographic evidence of consolidation.
- Slowly advance to full weight bearing in CAM boot over the next 6 weeks until patient can be fitted for custom shoes.
- Repeat radiographs every 2 weeks until Charcot stabilized and fully transitioned into a custom shoe.
- Follow-up every 6 months with repeat weight-bearing radiographs.
- Patients seen every 6 to 8 weeks in high-risk foot clinic for surveillance and callus care with nail trimming.

DURABLE MEDICAL EQUIPMENT

Durable medical equipment devices should be considered from day 1. Physicians should be familiar with the use of walkers, knee scooters, wheelchairs, crutches,

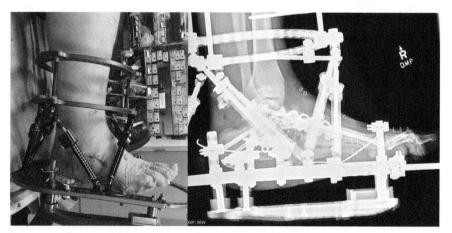

Fig. 7. Use of external fixation to protect the internal fixation.

I-walkers, bedside commodes, hospital beds, charcot restraint orthotic walker (CROW) boots, and custom shoes to best meet the needs of each patient. Ability to maintain nonweight bearing or minimal weight bearing is a critical part of achieving success in Charcot patients. A deformity can only be reduced and maintained if given the proper off-loading. Working with patients and family to attain these items promptly early on can be a deciding factor of a deformity being prevented or maintained. The authors' general surgical approach is to reconstruct and stabilize with the intent of transitioning into custom shoe gear. In general, the authors try to avoid use of a CROW boot in favor of custom shoe gear because of the overall low compliance with use of a CROW boot.

SUMMARY

In conclusion, the authors feel that aggressive treatment of the Charcot foot is crucial not only to their patients' long-term management of their deformity but also to their quality and length of life. Knowing that limb amputation carries with it known mortality risk within the following few years, simple logic supports Charcot reconstruction to delay death. Charcot is a dynamic process that challenges foot and ankle surgeons on many levels. Applying basic surgical principles and utilizing a team approach are critical in the successful management of this destructive condition.

DISCLOSURES

Neither author has any disclosures.

REFERENCES

1. DiDomenico L, Flynn Z, Reed M. Treating Charcot arthropathy is a challenge—explaining why my treatment algorithm has changed. Clin Podiatr Med Surg 2018; 35:105–21.
2. Tseng CH, Chong CK, Tseng CP, et al. Mortality, causes of death and associated risk factors in a cohort of diabetic patients after lower-extremity amputation: a 6.5-year follow-up study in Taiwan. Atherosclerosis 2008;197:111–7.
3. Hambleton IR, Jonnalagadda R, Davis CR, et al. All-cause mortality after diabetes-related amputation in Barbados: a prospective case-control study. Diabetes Care 2009;32:306–7.
4. Lavery LA, Hunt NA, Ndip A, et al. Impact of chronic kidney disease on survival after amputation in individuals with diabetes. Diabetes Care 2010;33:2365–9.
5. Armstrong DA, Swerdlow MA, Armstrong AA, et al. Five year mortality and direct costs of care for people with diabetic foot complications are comparable to cancer. J Foot Ankle Res 2020;13(1):16.
6. Sohn MW, Stuck RM, Pinzur M, et al. Lower-extremity amputation risk after charcot arthropathy and diabetic foot ulcer. Diabetes Care 2010;33(1):98–100.
7. La Fontaine J, Lavery L, Jude E. Current concepts of Charcot foot in diabetic patients. Foot 2016;26:7–14.
8. Blume PA, Sumpio B, Schmidt B, et al. Charcot neuroarthropathy of the foot and ankle—diagnosis and management strategies. Clin Podiatr Med Surg 2014;31: 151–72.
9. Rogers LC, Frykberg RG. The Charcot foot. Med Clin North Am 2013;97:847–56.
10. Nielson DL, Armstrong DG. The natural history of Charcot's neuroarthropathy. Clin Podiatr Med Surg 2008;25:53–62.

11. Younis BB, Shahid A, Arshad R, et al. Charcot osteoarthropathy in type 2 diabetes persons presenting to specialist diabetes clinic at a tertiary care hospital. BMC Endocr Disord 2015;15:28.
12. Wukich DK, Crim BE, Frykberg RG, et al. Neuropathy and poorly controlled diabetes increase the rate of surgical site infection after foot and ankle surgery. J Bone Joint Surg Am 2014;96(10):832–9.
13. McCann L, Zhu S, Pollard JD, et al. Success and survivorship following charcot reconstruction: a review of 151 cases. J Foot Ankle Surg 2021;60(3):535–40.

Current Concepts in Achilles Tendon Ruptures

Varsha Salunkhe Ivanova, DPM[a],*,
Khanh Phuong Sieu Tong, DPM, MSc[a], Cristian Neagu, DPM[b],
Christy M. King, DPM[c,d]

KEYWORDS

- Early functional rehabilitation • Minimally invasive surgery • Percutaneous surgery
- Open repair

KEY POINTS

- Acute Achilles tendon ruptures can be treated either conservatively or surgically, both with functional rehabilitation and early range of motion.
- Conservative therapy has evolved from immobilization with strict non-weight-bearing protocol, to early functional rehabilitation with earlier weight-bearing.
- Surgical treatment approaches vary from percutaneous, minimally invasive, and open repair.
- Current literature discussing surgical treatment for ruptured tendons shows low incidence of complications and similar functional outcomes.

INTRODUCTION

Considered the strongest tendon in the body, the Achilles tendon (AT) has been shown to have the highest incidence of ruptures. This is attributed to an aging population, obesity, and participation in sporting activities.[1] Some studies have shown a close association between tendon degeneration, medications (ie, fluoroquinolones, local corticosteroids), and systemic disease.[2] The injury has a bimodal distribution with a peak occurring in young males (20–39 year olds) and a second peak in middle-aged patients (40–59 year olds). The tendon, often pathologic in nature, ruptures with a forced dorsiflexion moment on a plantarflexed ankle. Typically, the ruptured tendon can be diagnosed with a clinical examination and utilization of the Thompson sign.[3,4]

[a] Kaiser Permanente Foot and Ankle Surgery, 700 Lawrence Expressway, Santa Clara, CA 95051, USA; [b] Kaiser Permanente Santa Clara Foot and Ankle Surgery, 700 Lawrence Expressway, Santa Clara, CA 95051, USA; [c] Kaiser Permanente, Department of Foot & Ankle Surgery, 3600 Broadway, Clinic 17, Oakland, CA 94611, USA; [d] Kaiser San Francisco Bay Area Foot & Ankle Residency Program, Oakland, CA, USA
* Corresponding author. 700 Lawrence Expressway, Santa Clara, CA 95051.
E-mail address: varsha.ivanova@gmail.com

Clin Podiatr Med Surg 41 (2024) 153–168
https://doi.org/10.1016/j.cpm.2023.09.001
0891-8422/24/© 2023 Elsevier Inc. All rights reserved.

The goal of acute AT rupture treatment is to allow the tendon to heal in a shortened position to avoid overlengthening the tendon and loss of strength and propulsion. This can be accomplished either with nonsurgical or surgical intervention (minimally invasive or open repair), both with early functional rehabilitation. Either treatment option offers excellent functional outcome with overall low risks.

ETIOLOGY AND DIAGNOSIS

The most common mechanism of injury leading to an AT rupture is participation in sports or recreational activity.[5] In a retrospective study of the epidemiology of AT ruptures, Lemme and colleagues found that out of 854 AT ruptures, recreational activity or sports accounted for 81.9% of all injuries with basketball (42.6%), soccer (9.9%), and football (8.4%) being most common in males, whereas in female patients, the most common mechanism of injury was volleyball (15.2%), basketball (14.8%), followed by track and field, gymnastics, and running/hiking.[5]

AT ruptures occur with an initial propulsive force with the knee extended followed by rapid dorsiflexion or with aggressive dorsiflexion of a plantarflexed ankle. An acceleration–deceleration event has been described in a large percentage of sports injuries.[6] As many as 25% of injuries can be missed at the time of diagnosis.[6] Clinically, local swelling, bruising, a palpable gap, positive Thompson's test, and decreased ankle plantar flexion strength typically suffice for an accurate diagnosis. MRI or ultrasonography is not routinely performed to confirm the presence of an acute rupture, however, may be performed to confirm the extent or location of the rupture, evaluate gap distance, or assist in surgical planning in delayed or chronic injuries.

ANATOMY

The AT is the primary muscle that produces ankle plantar flexion and is located within the superficial posterior muscle compartment of the lower leg. It is composed of the medial and lateral heads of the gastrocnemius and soleus muscle. The larger and stronger medial head of the gastrocnemius originates from the supracondylar ridge and adductor tubercle of the popliteal surface of the femur, whereas the lateral head originates from the lateral epicondyle. Both heads share the popliteal ligament as an additional origin. The soleus muscle originates distal to the knee from the posterior proximal tibia and the proximal one-third fibula posteriorly. These muscle bellies come together to form the AT, with the soleus forming the deeper portion, approximately 5 to 6 cm proximal to the insertion at the calcaneal tuberosity. As the tendon traverses distally, the medial fibers rotate posteriorly and lateral fibers rotate laterally, with an overall 90° rotation beginning above the region where the soleus and gastrocnemius join. This places the gastrocnemius portion on the lateral and posterior aspect of the tendon.[7–9] The tendon is rounded approximately 4 cm proximal to the insertion and flattens as it expands into a cartilaginous soft tissue structure and attaches to the posterior surface of the middle one-third of the calcaneal tuberosity.

At the insertion point of the AT, the tendinous fibers insert to the calcaneus via Sharpey's fibers. The endotenon is continuous with the periosteum, and superficial fibers are continuous with the fibrous tissue of the calcaneus extending distally to join the plantar fascia.[8,10–13] **Fig. 1** details the anatomy of the AT and change in the orientation of the tendon fibers.[14]

The plantaris is present in 92% to 94% of people and is a short muscle arising from the posterior surface of the femur, just proximal to the lateral femoral condyle. It has a long tendon that traverses between the gastrocnemius and soleus muscles and

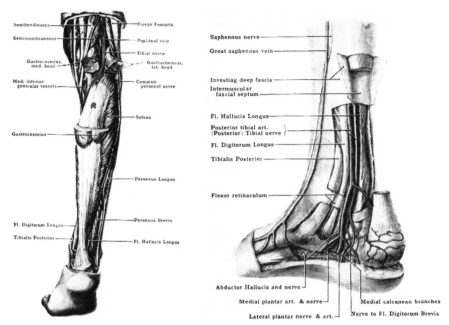

Fig. 1. Anatomy of the Achilles tendon and posterior ankle. (*From* Grant, J. C.Boileau. Grants Atlas of Anatomy. 5th ed.)

inserts into the medial border of the AT. In 6% to 8% of patients, this tendon separately inserts into the flexor retinaculum.[8]

Unlike most tendons, the AT is void of a tendinous sheath but is enclosed in a peritenon. This sheath is continuous proximally with crural fascia and distally with calcaneal periosteum. The peritenon is composed of connective tissue consisting of collagen type I, III, IV, and V, allows for gliding, and provides vascularity to the tendon.[8,15]

Considerations: Vascularity

Vascularity to the tendon is taken into account when considering the location of the rupture as well as for surgical planning. Historically, understanding of the vascular supply to the AT originated from Langergren's 1958 study, which designated the site of most frequent ruptures as a "watershed area."[16] The presence of this ischemic zone was believed to lead to tissue weakness and propensity for rupture. This theory was almost immediately challenged by Hastad who found continuous flow throughout the tendon.[17,18] A careful analysis of the AT shows that it receives its blood supply from different sources depending on anatomic location. Proximally, at the myotendinous junction, blood vessels from the surrounding tissues provide majority of vascularization, whereas the peritenon has been found to provide the circulation to the midportion of the AT. The distal one-third draws its blood supply from the blood vessels that supply the tendon–bone junction. Despite originating from three different anatomic locations, the overall blood supply to the AT is continuous in a longitudinal matter without actually penetrating the tendon fibers themselves.

A closer look by Yepes and colleagues at the skin and subcutaneous tissues of 10 cadaver legs found consistency within the blood supply to the AT.[19] They identified three vascular zones. The medial vascular zone, anatomically located between the posterior medial border of the tendon and posterior border of the medial malleolus, was found to be supplied by the posterior tibial artery via three or four perforating vessels and be significantly denser than the posterior zone. The lateral vascular zone, located between the posterior lateral border of the AT and posterior border of the lateral malleolus, was noted to have its peritenon and skin circulatory status provided by the peroneal artery and in 30% of specimens by recurrent branch of the peroneal artery. Similarly, the density in this region was greater than the posterior region. Finally, the posterior vascular zone, located directly over the AT, obtains its blood supply directly from perforating arteries and arterioles originating in the subcutaneous tissue and posterior peritenon. Aside from providing a clearer look at the vascular supply to the AT, their study made recommendations for incision placement during open AT repairs: Surgeons should favor either a medial incision located at least 1 cm medial to the AT or lateral incision with an associated risk of sural nerve injury. A straight posterior incision should be avoided given significant paucity of blood vessels, which may subsequently lead to a potential increase in wound complications.

If, as described above, the vascular supply to the AT is not compromised anatomically, are there other factors leading to potential ruptures? Under normal circumstances, physical activity produces an increase in metabolic demand characterized by cardiovascular redistribution of blood flow secondary to local vasodilation, which acts as a feedforward mechanism for exercise hyperemia.[17] Previous studies have shown that normal regulation of blood flow to skeletal muscle is age-dependent and thought to be a function of vascular stiffness and poor functioning of this feed forward mechanism.[20] Wezenbeek and colleagues have confirmed what other studies have already shown, a lower increase in blood flow in the 40- to 55-year-old group versus the younger cohort post-exercise, which can lead to decreased tensile strength with potential for structural weakness and poor healing potential.[21]

Considerations: Tendon Quality

Under normal circumstances, the AT is composed of multiple parallel bundles of type I collagen. Multiple fibrils are linked in succession to achieve the length of the tendon. This arrangement requires transfer of stress among individual units. In their findings, Jacobs and colleagues performed biopsies of ruptured ATs and found diffuse fibrosis, degenerative tendinous changes, and areas of longitudinal clefts due to fiber dissociation.[22] Their findings are consistent with previously published studies that showed that preexisting symptoms and degenerative changes in the AT can contribute to partial or complete rupture in injuries. Recent studies have, however, shown that chronic tendon changes are absent in approximately 25% of Achilles ruptures.[23] Type I collagen makes up 95% of the uninjured tendon fibers, whereas an injured tendon initially heals with type III collagen in injured, leading to less resistance to tensile forces and potentially higher rates of re-rupture.[24]

Considerations: Gap Distance

Gap distance defined as the distance between the ruptured tendon ends and can be used to guide treatment decisions and outcomes. In the literature, gap distance is most commonly measured using ultrasound because it can be measured with the ankle in a fully plantarflexed position.[25] In 2020, Yassin and colleagues assessed whether the size of tendon gap measured in maximum plantar flexion affects patient-reported outcomes following AT rupture treated with functional rehabilitation.[25] With a cohort of 82 patients, they found that increasing gap size over 5 mm predicts lower patient-reported outcomes, as measured by the Achilles Tendon Rupture Score. They concluded that a tendon gap greater than 5 mm may be a useful predictor in physically demanding individuals, and a tendon gap greater than 10 mm for those with low physical demand. On the other hand, Mubark and colleagues conducted a prospective case series ($n = 56$) with the gap distance measured with the ankle in neutral position.[26] By using AT gap measured in neutral position using ultrasound, re-rupture rates and outcome scores did not correlate with the size of the tendon gap. The results of these studies support that the ultrasound measured gap distance should be measured in maximum plantar flexion and can help influence potential outcomes and rate of re-rupture.

TREATMENT

Acute AT ruptures can be treated conservatively or with surgery. Conservative management of AT rupture has evolved from prolonged cast immobilization to utilization of early functional rehabilitation.[27] Surgical treatment has also evolved from long incisions to minimally invasive and percutaneous approaches.[28,29] The first article to compare conservative and surgical treatment was published by Jacobs and colleagues in 1978 who found superior functional outcomes in the operative group with plantar flexion force as compared with the nonoperative group; however, there was a paradigm shift with the publication of the early functional rehabilitation protocol with or without surgery by Willits and colleagues.[22,27]

Regardless of the treatment method, recent studies have shown that Soleus atrophy leading to loss of end-range plantar flexion torque is a common and persistent problem after AT ruptures, which will affect a patient's return to normal physical activity.[30] This finding was mirrored by Hodgens who found that Women's National Basketball Association (WNBA) players experience significant decrease in performance following AT rupture compared with preinjury level with 41.2% of players that return to the sport failing to play for more than one season and 23.5% of players failing to return to the sport following the injury.[31] Ultimately, the decision for conservative and surgical treatment will depend on multiple factors.

CONSERVATIVE TREATMENT

Conservative management of AT rupture previously involved prolonged cast immobilization, which is successful due to the tendon's ability to heal spontaneously in the position it is in, especially when tendon ends that are well opposed in a plantarflexed ankle are healthy and not pathologic.[32,33] However, side effects of prolonged immobilization are calf muscle atrophy and ankle joint stiffness to name a few. Deng and colleagues performed a large systematic review and meta-analysis of randomized controlled trials (RCTs) and found a re-rupture rate in the surgical group of 3.7% and nonsurgical group of 9.8%.[34] Of the nonsurgical group, approximately 30% were immobilized in a non-weight-bearing boot for 8 to 10 weeks.[34] Early weight-bearing in conjunction with functional rehabilitation has further been shown to have improved rates of re-rupture to that of prolonged non-weight-bearing of 3% and 5%, respectively.[35] Furthermore, the most of the re-ruptures have been found to take place within the first 12 weeks of surgery.[36]

Functional rehabilitation, which involves 2 to 3 weeks of cast immobilization, followed by controlled early weight-bearing, range of motion, and strengthening, helps to minimize these potential side effects. Several researchers have explored outcomes following a more functional rehabilitation protocol.[27] Willits and colleagues performed the first large RCT that compared outcomes of operative versus nonoperative treatment of acute AT ruptures.[27] Their study included 144 patients (118 males), with a mean age of 40.4 ± 8.8 years; 72 patients were treated operatively, and 72 patients were treated nonoperatively. Patients in the operative treatment group were treated in an open approach with Krackow-type stitch and plantarflexed splint. Both groups were treated with an initial non-weight-bearing plantarflexed splint for 2 weeks (either from day of injury or day of surgery), then transitioned to a walking boot with a 3 cm heel lift, similar to protocol outlined in **Table 1**. Researchers followed patients for 2 years and analyzed the outcomes including: re-rupture rate, strength range of motion, calf circumference, and Leppilahti score, a disease-specific functional outcome measure.[3] There was no statistically significant difference between the two groups, suggesting conservative therapy with the additional of functional rehabilitation for acute AT ruptures is an appropriate treatment alternative to surgical repair. More recently, a large systematic study of RCTs compared the functional outcomes of early controlled motion and weight-bearing (<3 weeks of rupture) and immobilization and delayed weight-bearing; their results found no statistically significant differences between re-rupture rate, return to sport/ work, and heel-rise work.[6] Almost 20 years ago, the Cochrane review published in 2004, showed the risk of re-rupture for surgical versus conservatively treated patients to be 3.5% and 12.6%, respectively.[38] However, in more recent studies, the re-rupture rate was found to be lower to around 2% to 3% with decreased period of cast immobilization and early functional rehabilitation.[27,39]

Nonoperative early functional rehabilitation treatment has been implemented in athletes and found to have a higher rate of return to pre-injury activity level in those with a lower pre-injury activity level.[40] In a study comparing pre-injury high-level activity (participation in competitive or recreational sports), and low-level activity (light/heavy labor, gymnastics, low-impact jogging/cycling), 67% of patients were able to return to their pre-injury high-level activity.[34] Functional outcomes including calf circumference, one-legged hop, and loss of power were not found to be statistically significantly different in both groups. In their findings, Deng and colleagues and Willits and colleagues found no statistically significant differences in incidence of deep vein thrombosis in surgically and conservatively treated groups.[27,34] At Kaiser Permanente Northern California, a modified early functional rehabilitation protocol was developed in conjunction with podiatry and physical therapy to optimize patient education and help to support return to activity (see **Table 1**).

SURGICAL TREATMENT

Surgical treatment for acute tendon rupture repair includes newer techniques such as percutaneous repair and minimally invasive surgery as well as the classic open repair. The goal of surgical repair is to anatomically reapproximate the ruptured tendon ends with a suture material to aid in regaining the appropriate length and tension.

PERCUTANEOUS REPAIR AND MINIMALLY INVASIVE SURGERY

Percutaneous AT repair was developed as early as 1977 by Ma and Griffith as an alternative to open procedures, which led to high risk of complications.[28] The initial percutaneous approach described involves six stab incisions (approximately 1 cm long) and was able to reduce skin incision size. However, it was initially associated with a high rate of re-rupture and nerve injury given lack of suturing under direct visualization. Utilization of the Ma and Griffith percutaneous repair led to sural nerve palsy in as many as 60% of the patients; however, later studies reported significantly lower rate of sural nerve complications at approximately 7%.[28,41] This has been primarily attributed to an increase in surgeon experience as well as development of surgical jigs, which make the surgical steps more predictable.

Modifications to the technique occurred in 1996 by Assal who developed a device that allowed visualization of the rupture site via small incisions (approximately

Table 1
The Kaiser Permanente Northern California modified early functional rehabilitation protocol

Phase I: Immediate Post-Injury Period (0–2 to 3 wk)

Rehabilitation goals	Protect tendon repair
	Reduce swelling, minimize pain
	Patient education
	Keep your leg up and elevated when sitting or lying down
	Do not put weight on the injured side
	Do not pivot on your injured side
Weight-bearing restrictions and precautions	Weight-bearing restrictions and precautions
	Weight-bearing status: Cast for 2–3 wk, strict non-weight-bearing
	Showering: Keep the cast clean and dry. You should cover it with a secure plastic wrap, so it does not get wet.
	Stairs: When climbing stairs, make sure you are leading with the non-injured side. It can be a safe alternative to go up and down the stairs on your buttocks.
Intervention	Swelling management: Ice, compression, elevation
	Cardio: upper body ergometer
Criteria to progress	2–3 wk

Phase II: Intermediate Post-Injury Period (2 to 3–6 wk)

Rehabilitation goals	Continue to protect the tendon repair while allowing for early range of motion to decrease adhesions
Weight-bearing restrictions	Weight-bearing status: Protected weight-bearing in the walking boot with ~3 × 5/16 heel lifts with crutch assistance. Heel lift height may vary per person.
	Sleeping: Keep the boot on at night when sleeping
	Showering: Use shower chair
	Stairs: When climbing or going downstairs, make sure you are leading with the uninjured side
Additional interventions	Swelling control: Ice, compression, elevation
	Cardio: upper body ergometer
	Scar management (if surgically corrected)
	Massage incision site
	You can apply topical scar treatments like vitamin E oil, Mederma cream (available in pharmacies), or silicon impregnated bandages (ie, Scar away or Mepiform available online)
	Range of motion/mobility
	Active range of motion plantar flexion, inversion, eversion, dorsiflexion from maximum plantar flexion to neutral (do not dorsiflex past neutral)
	Strengthening
	Hip and knee strengthening
	3-way hip
	Short/long arc quads
	Prone hamstring curls
	Open chain core
Criteria to progress	6 wk
	No wound complications
	Dorsiflexion to neutral

(continued on next page)

Table 1 *(continued)*	
Phase III: Late Post-Injury Period (6–8 wk)	
Rehabilitation goals	Start progression of weight-bearing without the boot increase dorsiflexion range of motion Safely progress strengthening Promote proper movement patterns Avoid post-exercise pain and swelling Avoid activities that produce pain at injured site
Weight-bearing restrictions	Weight-bearing status: Protected weight-bearing in the walking boot Week 6: Remove first heel lift Week 7: Remove second and third heel lifts Week 8: Start walking without the boot in supportive shoe Sleeping: You no longer need to sleep with the boot on

Additional interventions (continue with phase II interventions)	Cardio: Bike, swimming, water aerobics
	Scar management: Cross-friction massage incision site as needed
	Range of motion and mobility
	  Gentle calf stretching, non-weight-bearing
	  Ankle mobilizations, as needed
	Strengthening
	  Ankle dorsiflexion, plantar flexion, inversion, eversion with resistance band
	  Progress to weight-bearing hip/knee strengthening by week 8
	  Bridges, squats, step ups
	Neurologic re-education/proprioception
	  Static balance progression

Criteria to progress	Decrease in swelling and pain after exercise Dorsiflexion active range of motion to at least 5 Single leg stance for 30 s
Phase IV: Transitional Post-Injury Period (9–12 wk)	
Rehabilitation goals	Achieve full dorsiflexion range of motion Safely progress calf strengthening Promote proper movement patterns Avoid post-exercise pain and swelling

Additional interventions (continue with phase II–III interventions as needed)	Cardio: Bike, swimming, water aerobics, elliptical machine
	Range of motion and mobility
	  Calf stretching in weight-bearing
	  Ankle mobilizations, as needed
	Strengthening
	  Initiate heel raise progression, concentric and eccentric
	  Functional movements
	    Squats à single leg squat
	    Lunges (forward, lateral, reverse)
	    Step ups, step downs
	  Neurologic re-education and proprioception
	  Dynamic balance progression

Criteria to progress/return to impact training	Dorsiflexion range of motion equal to the contralateral side Ten repetitions of straight leg (SL) heel raise through 85% range of motion (contralateral side)

(continued on next page)

Table 1 (continued)	
Phase V: Early Return to Sport Period (3–5 mo)	
Rehabilitation goals	Maintain full range of motion Initiate plyometric program Safely initiate sport specific training program Avoid post-exercise pain and swelling

Additional interventions (continue with phase II–IV interventions)	Cardio: Bike, swimming, elliptical, running
	Plyometrics
	  Partial body weight with shuttle press
	  1. Bilateral hops
	  2. Alternating hops
	  3. Single leg hops
	  Frontal plane on land
	  4. Bilateral side to side
	  5. Single leg side to side
	  6. Skaters
	  Sagittal plane on land
	  7. Bilateral hops in place, forward/backward
	  8. Single leg hops in place, forward backward
	  9. Box jumps

Criteria to progress/return to run criteria	Single leg standing heel raise test: 90% Limb Symmetry Index (10 incline1 rep:2 s rate for 60 s, no. of reps performed) Single leg hop for distance 90% Limb Symmetry Index Single leg squat 45, 10 reps with good form
Phase VI: Unrestricted Return to Sport Period (6 mo)	
Rehabilitation goals	Safely return to sport

Additional interventions (continue with phase II–V interventions as needed)	Sport-specific agility and plyometric training
	  Examples:
	    Lateral shuffle, grapevine
	    Backwards running
	    Shuttle run
	    Sport cord drills
	    Ladder drills
	    T-agility
	    Box drill
	    Zig-zag run
	    Cutting and pivoting

Criteria to progress/return to unrestricted sport	Drop countermovement jump Limb Symmetry Index 90% (vertical drop from standard stair height of 20 cm) Ability to complete one repetition declined heel raise set at 20˙

Courtesy of Christy King, DPM and Kaillin Collins, DPT, Kaiser Permanente, Oakland, CA.[37]

5 cm long) and more precise suturing techniques led to a reduced risk for wound complications and rates of infection.[42] This is known as a mini open repair. Gatz and colleagues performed a multi-study analysis including 25 level I–III studies that only reported quantitative data under the outcomes of interest.[29] In their study, they found that compared with open repair, the minimally invasive surgical group had a shorter surgical duration, a lower rate of postoperative wound necrosis (0.38% vs 2.23% with open repair), superficial infection (0.19% vs 2.55% with open repair), and deep infection (2.20% vs 5.11% with open repair) and also experienced less scar tissue

with lesions (0.86% vs 4.57% with open repair). Similarly, no statistically significant differences were noted among the open and minimally invasive surgical approach with regard to postoperative re-rupture rates (2.10% vs 2.38% with open repair). Overall, compared with an open approach, visualization is limited with a percutaneous and minimally invasive approach, leading to higher risk of sural nerve injury; however, wound healing complications and re-rupture rates are comparable in more recent research.[43]

OPEN REPAIR

Open AT repair is used less than before with the advent of both early functional rehabilitation as well as percutaneous or minimally invasive approaches. Potential risks reported with the open approach include surgical site infection, wound dehiscence, and sural nerve injury. Although older studies reported higher rates of infection, wound dehiscence, and sural nerve injury, more recent studies have shown the risks to be significantly lower, allowing surgeons to reconsider the open approach.[44] Yamaguchi reported that despite an unchanged incidence of AT ruptures in Japan, 70% of patients underwent open surgical repair of their ruptures from 2010 to 2017.[44]

Multiple RCTs compare surgical and nonsurgical treatment options with recommendations dependent on chronicity of the studies. Pre-2005 RCTs reported a higher re-rupture rate with the conservative group, but despite higher rates of skin and neural entrapment complications recommended surgical repair.[45,46] Later studies showed that incorporation of early range of motion and weight-bearing led to similar re-rupture rates, calf circumference, functional outcomes, and strength.[47] In a recent retrospective study evaluating tendon length after operative or nonoperative treatment of AT ruptures, no statistically significant difference was found at a 1-year follow-up.[48] **Fig. 2**A shows a minimally plantarflexed ankle at rest and a palpable dell in the case of an AT rupture. **Fig. 2**B shows the results of open repair of the AT with the foot in more plantarflexed position at rest.

Historically, the Bunnell suture was reported to be superior, whereas the Krackow was associated with a higher potential of damage to the tendon secondary to increased strangulation and potential reduction of vascular supply.[49,50] It was also shown to be more technically difficult on the surgeon. Recent studies assessed the biomechanics of the sutures and found the double Bunnell to be the most resistant and also have the lowest degree of tendon elongation at the level of the rupture. Similar results with regard to resistance were noted in the Kraków suture; however, it resulted in greater elongation of the tendon.[51] **Figs. 3** and **4** show the frayed tendon ends of an acute AT rupture open repair and reapproximation of the tendon ends with

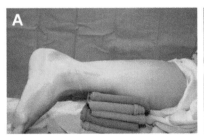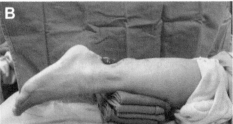

Fig. 2. (*A, B*) Acute ruptured Achilles tendon is notable for a posterior dell and dorsiflexed ankle joint at rest. Post-tendon open tendon rupture repair shows a plantarflexed ankle at rest.

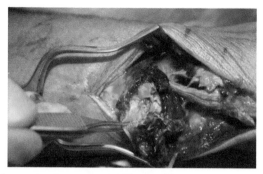

Fig. 3. Frayed tendon ends of an acute Achilles tendon rupture.

nonabsorbable suture in a Krakow fashion. Despite the close opposition of tendon ends, the weakest point of the surgical repair rests with the surgical knots. Specialized suturing techniques were developed by Bunnell, Kessler, and Krackow with good results **(Fig. 5)**.[49,50,52,53]

Soroceanu and colleagues performed a meta-analysis of 10 RCTs and compared an operatively treated group (either open or minimally invasive techniques) and nonoperatively treated group (with or without functional rehabilitation with early range of motion).[36] Their data demonstrated similar rates of re-rupture with operative and nonoperative with functional rehabilitation (risk difference 1.7%, $P = .45$). Furthermore, there was no statistically significant difference between the nonoperative and operative groups regarding calf circumference, strength, and functional outcome. Patients treated operatively are found to return to work sooner than those treated conservatively.[47]

CHRONIC RUPTURE TREATMENT

Although the best treatment approach to acute Achilles ruptures is debatable, it is well accepted in the literature that open repair of AT injuries is indicated in the setting of chronic ruptures as well as acute injuries in the young, healthy, athletic patient. In most cases, however, the choice of surgical procedure is surgeon and patient-dependent. The goal of management of a chronic Achilles rupture is to bring the injured tendon ends in close apposition, restore normal length–tension to improve

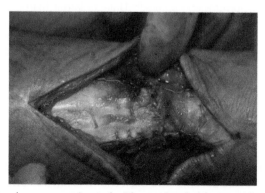

Fig. 4. Ruptured tendon reapproximated with nonabsorbable suture in Krakow fashion.

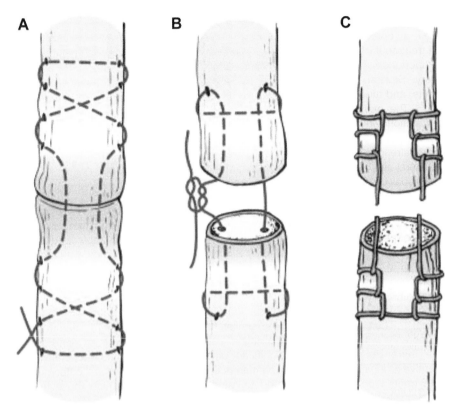

Fig. 5. Tendon repair techniques. (*A*) Modified Bunnell technique. (*B*) Kessler technique. (*C*) Krackow technique. (*From* Coughlin MJ Saltzman CL Anderson RB. Mann's Surgery of the Foot and Ankle. Ninth ed. Philadelphia PA: Saunders/Elsevier; 2014.)

strength with an early return to normal function while maintaining complications to a minimum.

The open surgical repair technique for chronic ruptures depends on several factors, including age of the AT injury, time from injury to surgery, size of the defect, and intra-operative findings.[54] In most cases, if the defect between measures less than 3 cm, an end-to-end repair can be performed using a multi-strand, long chain ultra-high molecular weight braided polyethylene suture.[55] Defects larger than 3 cm may require a gastrocnemius recession or myotendinous flaps to increase the length of the muscle and close the rupture gap. Techniques using flexor hallucis longus or plantaris tendon have been described to augment the repair and improve local blood supply without functional deficiencies distally at the digital level.[55,56]

Open repair of the AT continues to remain a good option in the setting of an acute rupture and the recommended form of treatment for chronic ruptures. Historically, studies have shown a lower rate of re rupture as compared with the conservatively managed patients, which was offset with employment of functional rehabilitation programs aimed at early range of motion and weight-bearing. Surgeons must however take into consideration the possible complications commonly associated with surgery such as superficial and deep infection occurring in 2.6% and 5.1% of patients, respectively.[29] Surgically treated patients have been shown to have an early return to weight-bearing and return to work.

SUMMARY

There is an ongoing debate between the risks and benefits of conservative and operative treatment of AT ruptures. Regardless of treatment selected, research supports the importance of functional rehabilitation with weight-bearing whether with or without surgery. Several comparative studies have been published that review the risks, benefits, and functional outcomes of operatively and nonoperatively treated AT ruptures.[29] The main complications compared include rates of re-rupture, infection, and functional outcomes. Functional outcomes after an AT rupture may be poor due to the risk of tendon elongation, inevitable muscle weakness, and decreased push off strength. Complications in the open repair such as superficial and deep infections, sural nerve injury, and re-rupture are significantly improved with new percutaneous repair techniques. Overall, recent literature shows a similar rate of re-rupture between the surgical and nonsurgical treatment groups if a functional rehabilitation protocol with early range of motion and weight bearing is performed.

CLINICS CARE POINTS

- Early diagnosis and treatment of Achilles tendon ruptures are imperative to avoid complications of chronic Achilles tendon ruptures.
- Recent literature shows similar rates of re-rupture with conservative or surgical treatment.
- Weight-bearing functional rehabilitation plays an important role in the recovery after Achilles tendon injuries, treated with or without surgery.

DISCLOSURES

The authors have nothing to disclose regarding conflict of interest or commercial relationship related to the content of this work.

REFERENCES

1. Raikin SM, Garras DN, Krapchev PV. Achilles tendon injuries in a United States population. Foot Ankle Int 2013;34(4):475–80.
2. Järvinen TAH, Kannus P, Maffulli N, et al. Achilles tendon disorders: etiology and epidemiology. Foot Ankle Clin 2005;10(2):255–66.
3. Leppilahti J, Orava S. Total Achilles tendon rupture. A review. Sports Med 1998; 25(2):79–100.
4. Maffulli N. Current concepts in the management of subcutaneous tears of the Achilles tendon. Bull Hosp Jt Dis 1998;57(3):152–8.
5. Lemme NJ, Li NY, DeFroda SF, et al. Epidemiology of Achilles tendon ruptures in the United States: athletic and nonathletic injuries from 2012 to 2016. Orthop J Sports Med 2018;6(11). 2325967118808238.
6. Gobbi A, Espregueira-Mendes J, Lane JG, et al. Bio-orthopaedics: a new approach. Berlin, Germany: Springer; 2017.
7. Barfred T. Experimental rupture of the Achilles tendon. Comparison of various types of experimental rupture in rats. Acta Orthop Scand 1971;42(6):528–43.
8. O'Brien M. The anatomy of the Achilles tendon. Foot Ankle Clin 2005;10(2): 225–38.
9. Benjamin M, Evans EJ, Copp L. The histology of tendon attachments to bone in man. J Anat 1986;149:89–100.

10. Kvist M. Achilles tendon overuse injuries: a clinical and pathophysiological study in athletes with special reference to Achilles Paratenonitis. 1991.

11. Allenmark C. Partial Achilles tendon tears. Clin Sports Med 1992;11(4):759–69.

12. Kvist M. Achilles tendon injuries in athletes. Sports Med 1994;18(3):173–201.

13. Jones FW. Structure and Function as Seen in the Foot.; 1949.

14. Boileau GJC. Grant's atlas of anatomy. Baltimore, MD: Williams & Wilkins; 1972. p. 318–21.

15. Schepsis AA, Jones H, Haas AL. Achilles tendon disorders in athletes. Am J Sports Med 2002;30(2):287–305.

16. Lagergren C, Lindbom A, Soderberg G. Hypervascularization in chronic inflammation demonstrated by angiography; angiographic, histopathologic, and microangiographic studies. Acta Radiol 1958;49(6):441.

17. Fadel PJ. Reflex control of the circulation during exercise. Scand J Med Sci Sports 2015;25(suppl 4):74–82.

18. Hastad K, Larsson LG, Lindholm A. Clearance of radiosodium after local deposit in the Achilles tendon. Acta Chir Scand 1959;116:251–5.

19. Yepes H, Tang M, Geddes C, et al. Digital vascular mapping of the integument about the Achilles tendon. J Bone Joint Surg Am 2010;92(5):1215–20.

20. CMJr Hearon, Dinenno FA. Regulation of skeletal muscle blood flow during exercise in ageing humans. J Physiol 2016;594(8):2261–73.

21. Wezenbeek E, Willems T, Mahieu N, et al. The role of the vascular and structural response to activity in the development of achilles tendinopathy: a prospective study. Am J Sports Med 2018;46(4):947–54.

22. Jacobs D, Martens M, Van Audekercke R, et al. Comparison of conservative and operative treatment of Achilles tendon rupture. Am J Sports Med 1978;6(3): 107–11.

23. Park YH, Kim TJ, Choi GW, et al. Achilles tendinosis does not always precede Achilles tendon rupture. Knee Surg Sports Traumatol Arthrosc 2019;27(10): 3297–303.

24. Tarantino D, Palermi S, Sirico F, et al. Achilles tendon rupture: mechanisms of injury, principles of rehabilitation and return to play. J Funct Morphol Kinesiol 2020;5(4). https://doi.org/10.3390/jfmk5040095.

25. Yassin M, Myatt R, Thomas W, et al. Does size of tendon gap affect patient-reported outcome following Achilles tendon rupture treated with functional rehabilitation? Bone Joint Lett J 2020;102-B(11):1535–41.

26. Mubark I, Abouelela A, Arya S, et al. Achilles tendon rupture: can the tendon gap on ultrasound scan predict the outcome of functional rehabilitation program? Cureus 2020;12(9):e10298.

27. Willits K, Amendola A, Bryant D, et al. Operative versus nonoperative treatment of acute Achilles tendon ruptures: a multicenter randomized trial using accelerated functional rehabilitation. J Bone Joint Surg Am 2010;92(17):2767–75.

28. Ma GW, Griffith TG. Percutaneous repair of acute closed ruptured achilles tendon: a new technique. Clin Orthop Relat Res 1977;128:247–55.

29. Gatz M, Driessen A, Eschweiler J, et al. Open versus minimally-invasive surgery for Achilles tendon rupture: a meta-analysis study. Arch Orthop Trauma Surg 2021;141(3):383–401.

30. Wenning M, Mauch M, Heitner A, et al. Midterm functional performance following open surgical repair of acute Achilles tendon rupture. Arch Orthop Trauma Surg 2022;142:1337–49.

31. Hodgens B, Geller J, Rizzo MG, et al. Performance outcomes after surgical repair of achilles tendon rupture in the women's national basketball association. Orthopaedic Journal of Sports Medicine 2021;9(9). 23259671211030473.

32. Bruns J, Kampen J, Kahrs J, et al. Achilles tendon rupture: experimental results on spontaneous repair in a sheep-model. Knee Surg Sports Traumatol Arthrosc 2000;8(6):364–9.

33. Lea RB, Smith L. Rupture of the achilles tendon. Nonsurgical treatment. Clin Orthop Relat Res 1968;60:115–8.

34. Deng S, Sun Z, Zhang C, et al. Surgical treatment versus conservative management for acute achilles tendon rupture: a systematic review and meta-analysis of randomized controlled trials. J Foot Ankle Surg 2017;56(6):1236–43.

35. Young SW, Patel A, Zhu M, et al. Weight-bearing in the nonoperative treatment of acute achilles tendon ruptures: a randomized controlled trial. J Bone Joint Surg Am 2014;96(13):1073–9.

36. Reito A, Logren HL, Ahonen K, et al. Risk factors for failed nonoperative treatment and rerupture in acute achilles tendon rupture. Foot Ankle Int 2018;39(6): 694–703.

37. King CM, Vartivarian M. Achilles tendon rupture repair: simple to complex. Clin Podiatr Med Surg 2023;40(1):75–96.

38. Khan RJ, Carey Smith RL. Surgical interventions for treating acute Achilles tendon ruptures. Cochrane Database Syst Rev 2010;9:CD003674.

39. Nilsson-Helander K, Silbernagel KG, Thomeé R, et al. Acute achilles tendon rupture: a randomized, controlled study comparing surgical and nonsurgical treatments using validated outcome measures. Am J Sports Med 2010;38(11): 2186–93.

40. Lerch TD, Schwinghammer A, Schmaranzer F, et al. Return to sport and patient satisfaction at 5-year follow-up after nonoperative treatment for acute achilles tendon rupture. Foot Ankle Int 2020;41(7):784–92.

41. Grassi A, Amendola A, Samuelsson K, et al. Minimally invasive versus open repair for acute achilles tendon rupture: meta-analysis showing reduced complications, with similar outcomes, after minimally invasive surgery. J Bone Joint Surg Am 2018;100(22):1969–81.

42. Assal M, Jung M, Stern R, et al. Limited open repair of Achilles tendon ruptures: a technique with a new instrument and findings of a prospective multicenter study. J Bone Joint Surg Am 2002;84(2):161–70.

43. Li Y, Jiang Q, Chen H, et al. Comparison of mini-open repair system and percutaneous repair for acute Achilles tendon rupture. BMC Musculoskelet Disord 2021;22(1):914.

44. Yamaguchi S, Kimura S, Akagi R, et al. Increase in achilles tendon rupture surgery in Japan. Orthopaedic Journal of Sports Medicine 2021;9(10).

45. Moller M, Movin T, Granhed H, et al. Acute rupture of tendon Achillis: a prospective randomised study of comparison between surgical and nonsurgical treatment. J Bone Joint Surg Br 2001;83:84.

46. Bhandari M, Guyatt G, Siddiqui F, et al. Treatment of acute Achilles tendon ruptures: a systematic overview and metaanalysis. Clin Orthop Relat Res 2002; 400:190–200.

47. Soroceanu A, Sidhwa F, Aarabi S, et al. Surgical versus nonsurgical treatment of acute Achilles tendon rupture: a meta-analysis of randomized trials. J Bone Joint Surg Am 2012;94(23):2136–43.

48. Cramer A, Rahdi E, Hansen MS, et al. No clinically relevant difference between operative and non-operative treatment in tendon elongation measured with the

Achilles tendon resting angle (ATRA) 1 year after acute Achilles tendon rupture. Knee Surg Sports Traumatol Arthrosc 2021;29(5):1617–26.

49. Krackow KA, Thomas SC, Jones LC. A new stitch for ligament-tendon fixation. Brief note. J Bone Joint Surg Am 1986;68(5):764–6.

50. Bunnell S, Boyes JH. Bunnell's surgery of the hand. Philadelphia, PA: J.P. Lippincott; 1970.

51. Manent A, Lopez L, Vilanova J, et al. Assessment of the resistance of several suture techniques in human cadaver achilles tendons. J Foot Ankle Surg 2017;56: 954–9.

52. Kessler I, Nissim F. Primary repair without immobilization of flexor tendon division within the digital sheath. An experimental and clinical study. Acta Orthop Scand 1969;40(5):587–601.

53. Coughlin MJ, Saltzman CL, Anderson RB. Mann's surgery of the foot and ankle. 9th edition. Philadelphia PA: Saunders/Elsevier; 2014.

54. Kuwada GT. An update on repair of achilles tendon rupture. acute and delayed. J Am Podiatr Med Assoc 1999;89(6):302–6.

55. Aktas S, Kocaoglu B, Nalbantoglu U, et al. End-to-end versus augmented repair in the treatment of acute Achilles tendon ruptures. J Foot Ankle Surg 2007;46(5): 336–40.

56. Maffulli N, Gougoulias N, Christidis P, et al. Primary augmentation of percutaneous repair with flexor hallucis longus tendon for Achilles tendon ruptures reduces tendon elongation and may improve functional outcome. Knee Surg Sports Traumatol Arthrosc 2023;31(1):94–101.

Batting Cleanup
Revision of Surgical Misadventure

Jessica Lickiss, DPM*, Glenn Weinraub, DPM

KEYWORDS

- Revision surgery • Malunion • Nonunion • Deformity • Post operative complications

KEY POINTS

- Surgical complications are a part of every surgeon's practice.
- Handling surgical complications appropriately includes deciphering what portion of the preoperative, operative, or postoperative period resulted in the outcome.
- Setting realistic expectations with your patients and ensuring informed consent will allow for the best outcome.

INTRODUCTION

Surgical outcomes are dependent on a variety of factors, including appropriate patient selection, proper procedure selection, surgical execution, choice of fixation, postoperative protocol, and expectations set from the provider to the patient. Most pathologies in the foot and ankle have multiple choices for procedure and for the execution of hardware. Many surgical principles should always be considered to decrease the chance of complications. These include utilizing appropriate surgical technique and respecting how bone and soft tissues need to heal.[1,2]

Complications are a part of every surgeon's practice and learning how to discuss the unexpected outcome with a patient with humility, respect, and a plan for addressing the complication are important lessons to learn. "Good Surgical Judgment comes from experience, and experience comes from poor surgical judgment."[3] It can sometimes feel that you are always changing your practice based on your most recent complications. Handling surgical complications requires deciphering what portion of the patient's history/comorbidities, preoperative workup, surgery, or the postoperative period contributed to the outcome. Many times, there are multiple factors influencing the surgical results. The next step is deciding if operating again would benefit the patient or cause more harm, and what procedure would be appropriate. The last portion to consider is setting realistic expectations for the patient for their final

Orthopedics Department, Kaiser Permanente Santa Clara Residency Program, Kaiser Permanente GSAA, 2500 Merced Street, San Leandro, CA 94577, USA
* Corresponding author.
E-mail address: Jessica.lickiss@kp.org

Clin Podiatr Med Surg 41 (2024) 169–192
https://doi.org/10.1016/j.cpm.2023.06.006
0891-8422/24/© 2023 Elsevier Inc. All rights reserved.
podiatric.theclinics.com

outcomes. In many cases, revision surgery can improve a patient's pain or current scenario, but it may not be able to fully alleviate the symptoms they are experiencing or regain full function. Foot and ankle surgery may involve common complications such as infection, nerve damage, painful scar formation, bone healing, painful hardware, recurrent deformity, and pain. Complications can be related to the preoperative, intraoperative, and postoperative period. For the revision, it is important to identify factors that can be modified to ensure the patient has a better outcome with their revision surgery. This could include help from the patient's primary physician to optimize the patient's co-morbidities, education, nutritional changes, physical therapy, and assistive devices.[4–6] Finally, it is essential to manage patients' postoperative expectations and psyche, ensuring that patients fully understand all possible complications and potential for further surgery needed and where the pitfalls occurred in their last surgery.

Perioperative Points to Consider

Patient comorbidities can have a significant impact on surgical outcome. Wound complications and bone healing issues can arise from a patient's nutritional status, medications they are taking around the time of surgery, and overall health. Depending on the surgery and postoperative protocol, a patients' home and support system is also imperative for successful healing. Smoking cessation is critical for any surgeries requiring bone healing particularly in the foot and ankle.

Procedure selection is also critical to the patients' outcome. There are multiple procedures to address many of the common pathologies that we see in foot and ankle surgery. An honest discussion with the patient about their goals and their ability to do the recovery needed is critical for a good outcome.

CASE 1

47-year-old male with type 2 diabetes mellitus (DM), congestive heart failure (CHF), hypertension (HTN), psoriasis, and previous amphetamine use disorder sustained a bimalleolar ankle fracture dislocation. He was closed reduced in the emergency room and was subsequently taken to the operating room for fixation within 2 weeks by the orthopedics department. The patient missed his first postoperative visit and presented to clinic 4 weeks postop with swelling, edema and pain (**Fig. 1**). He presented in a shoe and said that his splint was bothersome, and he removed it prior to his first-week postoperative visit. His radiographs revealed malreduction of the medial malleolar fracture, widening of the medial clear space, lucency around syndesmotic screw and fibula hardware intact. Unfortunately, there were no direct postoperative films to see his position and reduction intra operatively (**Fig. 2**). It is imperative for everyone patient to have intra operative fluoroscopy imaging or direct postoperative films to show that the patient left the surgery in an appropriate position. He then presented to podiatry for second opinion for further surgery. The patient was noted to have profound neuropathy, and a frank discussion was had about attempting a revision and the high risk for wound complication or potential loss of limb. The patient was amenable to revision and agreed to be non-weight bearing after surgery. The patient underwent revision open reduction and internal fixation (ORIF). His medial malleolar fracture piece was too small to use direct screw fixation, so a hook plate was utilized instead with good purchase and reduction. As an alternative to consider, a tension band technique could have been used in lieu of this. A new fibular plate was placed to allow for two syndesmotic screws (**Figs. 3** and **4**). The patient had significant swelling in his leg during his surgery, so an incisional wound VAC was placed,

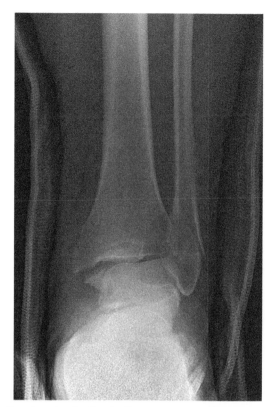

Fig. 1. Preop XR after closed reduction in the emergency room.

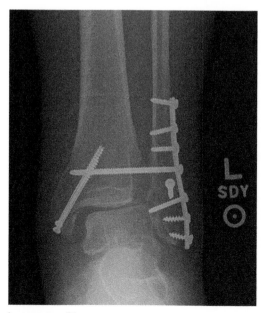

Fig. 2. Index procedure postop films.

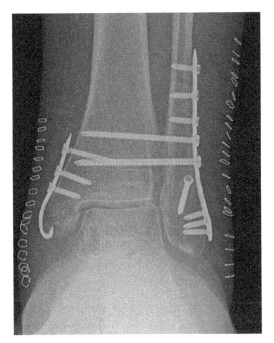

Fig. 3. Postop XR after revision surgery.

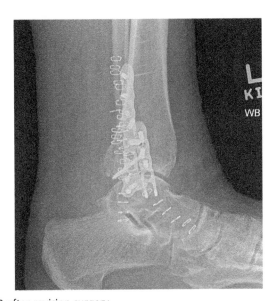

Fig. 4. Postop XR after revision surgery.

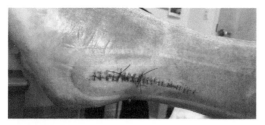

Fig. 5. Clinic image after revision surgery and removal of incisional VAC.

and he was seen within 1 week for a wound check. At this appointment, his incision appeared mildly macerated but overall healing well. Unfortunately, at 3 weeks postoperative, he dehisced a portion of his incision (**Figs. 5–7**). He underwent local wound care and a subsequent attempt at surgical closure, including the application of an integra graft. The patient continued to have swelling issues in his lower extremity related to a CHF exacerbation and he continued to have a hypergranular wound. His labs and scans indicated no evidence of osteomyelitis. He was referred to plastics who discussed potential surgery, however with his CHF and DM not well managed (HbA1C 10), they recommended local wound care. Within 3 month's time, the patient's syndesmotic screws subsequently started backing out (**Figs. 8 and 9**). He was taken to the operating room for an incision and drainage and removal of the screw with wound VAC application. To be complete, a bone biopsy and culture were sent and were negative for osteomyelitis. The wound VAC was used for a month. He was on oral antibiotics during this time period. His ankle hardware continued to remain stable, and he received nursing care to help with edema management as well as help from his primary physician to manage his overall health. With time, his incision did heal and total healing time took 1 year from the original injury. The patient's primary physician helped with managing his CHF and DM, and his wife helped with support during his nonweight-bearing portion of his postoperative recovery. This patient's compliance and neuropathy complicated his original outcome, and a larger construct was needed to provide the support necessary to heal. With his first surgery his medial malleolar fracture was likely never reduced appropriately, and hardware was never in the appropriate alignment across the fracture site. His associated complications were impacted by his edema issues and his comorbidities.

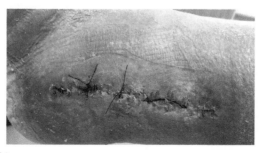

Fig. 6. Surgical dehiscence.

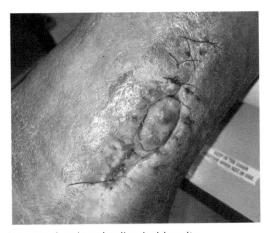

Fig. 7. Hypergranular wound and nonhealing incision site.

CASE 2

64-year-old female with a history of foot drop, traumatic brain injury, and rigid pes planus underwent surgery over 15 years prior to consultation with an attempted triple arthrodesis. The patient was noncompliant postoperatively because she was still caring for her children, and she developed a rigid valgus deformity with her foot resting abducted to her leg. She originally presented 3 years prior to the podiatry clinic with a fibula stress fracture due to the rigid valgus position of her foot and ankle. She presented to the clinic again and asked if she could undergo revision surgery since she was unable to wear a shoe because her foot is "pointing the wrong direction." At this point, her children were grown, and she had the time to recover appropriately. After a long discussion about potential issues with healing due to patient's age and comorbidities developed since her last surgery, the patient opted for an ankle

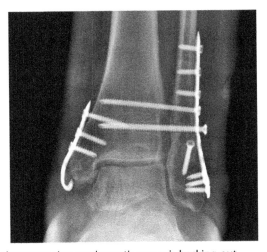

Fig. 8. Postop XR demonstrating syndesmotic screw is backing out.

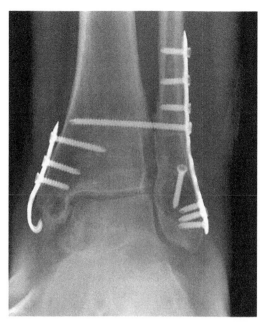

Fig. 9. Postop image after removal of syndesmotic screw and bone biopsy.

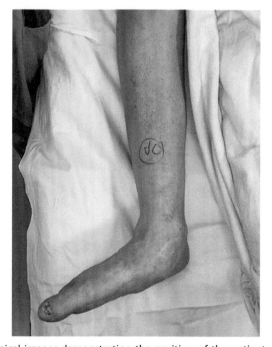

Fig. 10. Preop clinical images demonstrating the position of the patients foot to her leg.

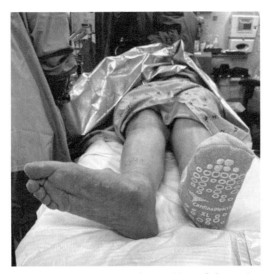

Fig. 11. Preop clinical images demonstrating the position of the patients foot to her leg.

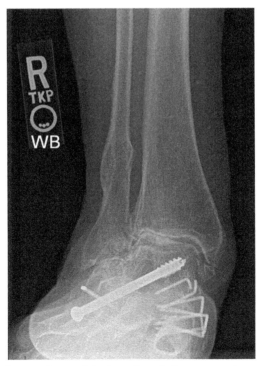

Fig. 12. Preop XRs from patients original rearfoot fusion surgery demonstrating hardware failure and valgus position.

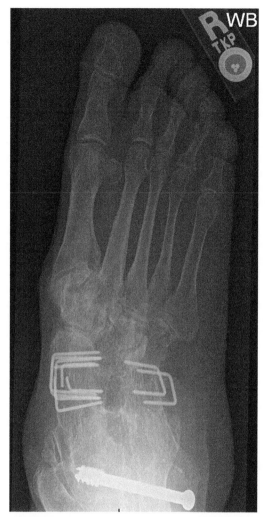

Fig. 13. Preop XRs from patients original rearfoot fusion surgery demonstrating hardware failure and valgus position.

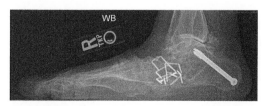

Fig. 14. Preop XRs from patients original rearfoot fusion surgery demonstrating hardware failure and valgus position.

arthrodesis with a revision of her rearfoot fusion in an attempt to get her foot plantigrade (**Figs. 10–14**).

Intraoperatively, the patient's bone quality was very soft, and her hardware was easy to remove both medially and laterally. Her calcaneal screw was left in place due to her bone quality, and it was elected to leave the subtalar joint fusion and heel in slight valgus with an attempt to adduct the forefoot on the rearfoot to establish a more plantigrade foot. This was done with the understanding that the overall position of her foot to her leg was more rectus and would allow her to ambulate better than before her surgery. An osteotomy or take down of her previous subtalar arthrodesis could have been performed with bone graft, however with her poor bone quality it was decided that there would be the minimal correction from doing this and posed another area for healing for her. An opening wedge was performed at her previous calcaneal cuboid (CC) fusion site with an iliac crest allograft with osteoinductive bone paste was placed and a closing wedge was performed at her previous talonavicular (TN) fusion site. This resulted in the forefoot and midfoot adducting on the rearfoot and finding a rectus position. Next, her ankle joint was prepped and then hardware was placed. Her original surgery involved using staples for her TN and CC fusion sites and one subtalar joint screw. For this surgery, more robust hardware was placed including plates and screws. Likely her original outcome resulted from compliance and from the fixation choices. Overall, her foot and ankle were in a rectus position. The patient is currently in regular supportive shoe gear with an Arizona brace and functioning well. She had no wound complications, and was happy with her final results. Reaching her goals, she is able to go grocery shopping again and travel with her husband which she had not been able to do for many years (**Figs. 15–17**).

CASE 3

48-year-old male with bilateral cavus feet with ankle instability. He underwent reconstruction bilaterally (on separate occasions spaced apart by 4 months), including a

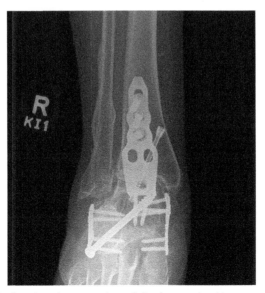

Fig. 15. Postop XRs showing the correction of the foot and ankle.

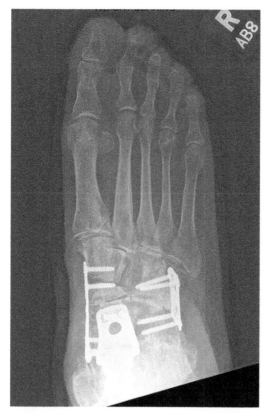

Fig. 16. Postop XRs showing the correction of the foot and ankle.

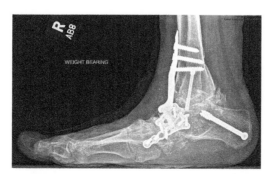

Fig. 17. Postop XRs showing the correction of the foot and ankle.

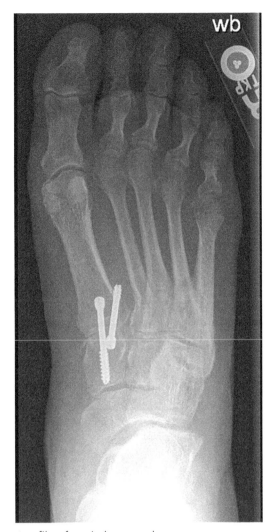

Fig. 18. Patients postop films from index procedure.

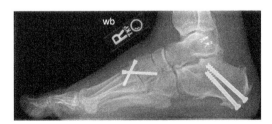

Fig. 19. Patients postop films from index procedure.

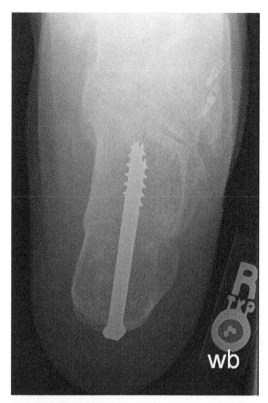

Fig. 20. Patients postop films from index procedure.

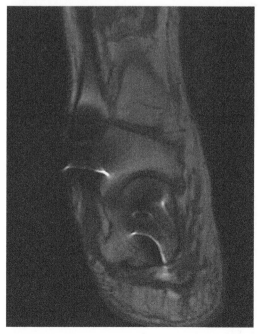

Fig. 21. Preoperative MRI that does demonstrate patients lateral coalition.

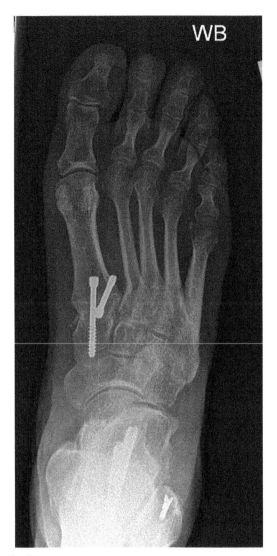

Fig. 22. Postoperative XRs.

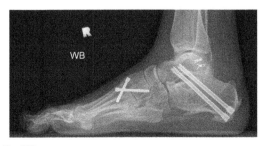

Fig. 23. Postoperative XRs.

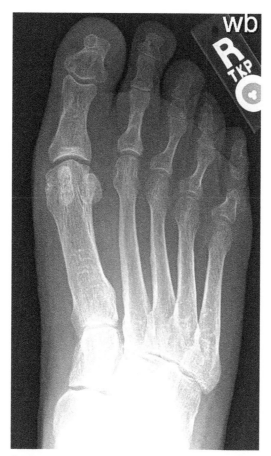

Fig. 24. Postop XRs from patients index procedure showing the aggressive resection of the proximal phalanx of the 5th toe.

Dwyer, Steindler stripping, dorsiflexory osteotomy first ray, ankle stabilization, and posterior tibial tendon transfer (**Figs. 18–20**). The patient was happy with his left foot results, but he felt that his right foot was similar to his position prior to surgery with pressure on the outside of the foot and ankle. In addition, he noticed a lump on the front of his lower leg with some weakness with dorsiflexion. The lump had appeared around 3 months postoperatively along with the change in dorsiflexion. The patient came to the clinic for second opinion around 4 months postop. On exam, his foot was loading in a varus position and the lump on his lower leg was mobile but firm. An MRI was obtained which revealed the lump was actually his posterior tibial tendon from his transfer surgery which had pulled from his tenodesis site and was stuck the transfer site at the interosseous membrane. The discussion with the patient included considering an attempt to transfer the tendon to his lateral cuneiform and perform a subtalar joint arthrodesis to allow for more control of the overall position of his hindfoot. His initial postoperative radiographs showed that his heel was corrected appropriately with the Dwyer and was in a rectus position, but his overall position during stance was still in varus. During surgery, it was identified that he had a coalition between his calcaneus and talus laterally with a full facet formed, causing

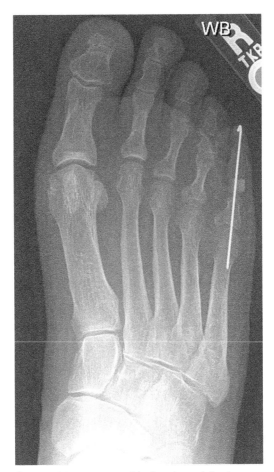

Fig. 25. Postop XRs from revision surgery with the pin and finals.

a boney block and the varus position (**Fig. 21**). His second surgery allowed for the facet to be removed and small wedge resection laterally to place the rearfoot into a rectus position to the ankle, and his PT tendon was reattached to the lateral cuneiform. The patient is currently doing well and working with physical therapy to regain strength in his leg after 2 large podiatric surgical recoveries for his right side. Now, his foot is hitting the ground in a rectus position with heel strike, and his posterior tibial tendon transfer continues to function well. This patient had no compliance issues, but instead, had aberrant anatomy that was not identified prior to his original surgery (**Figs. 22** and **23**).

CASE 4

65-year-old male with past medical history of lower back surgery had 5th toe arthroplasty 15 years prior to consultation for painful corn. His corn never recurred but his toe was completely floppy after the procedure. He had difficulty putting socks on as it would get caught easily. During the consultation options discussed included potential amputation versus attempt at reconstruction. During his reconstruction case,

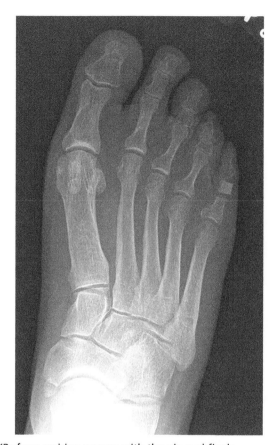

Fig. 26. Postop XRs from revision surgery with the pin and finals.

it was identified that all extensor and flexor tendons were cut and not repaired with his original procedure. He also had an aggressive resection of his proximal phalanx. It was opted to fashion a small graft from iliac crest allograft to fill the space and pin the toe. Originally, a screw was going to be placed, but due to the size of the graft and the small size of the toe, it was decided a pin would be a better option. The distal portion of the proximal phalanx was freshened with a saw with hopes for an arthrodesis, or at the very least, a pseudoarthrosis to provide toe stability. The remaining extensor tendon was reattached to the bone to provide some additional stability and scar formation. A skin plasty performed plantarly as a small ellipse of tissue at the metatarsophalangeal joint (MTPJ), was utilized to assist in keeping the toe in a rectus position. At 5 weeks, the pin was removed on accident at home prior to planned timing. The graft site created a pseudoarthrosis, and the patient was happy with the results and had a stable toe that he could easily put socks on and walk without issue. Overall, the success with the procedure was creating stability and increased length to the toe for a more normal position. An arthroplasty may have been the correct procedure for this patient, however with all tendons severed, there was no structural stability to the toe. With any procedure, it is important to consider the structural integrity provided by both the bone and soft tissues (**Figs. 24–27**).

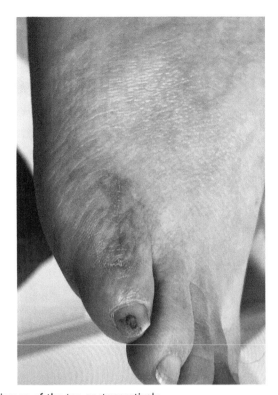

Fig. 27. Clinical image of the toe postoperatively.

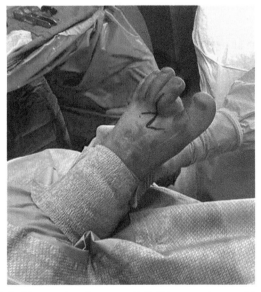

Fig. 28. Intra op clinical image showing second digit hammertoe, and incision planning for the Z plasty.

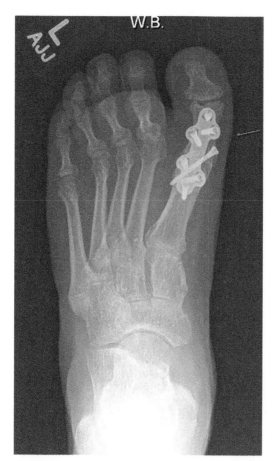

Fig. 29. Postop XRs from patients index procedure from outside the hospital.

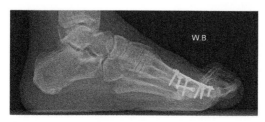

Fig. 30. Postop XRs from patients index procedure from outside the hospital.

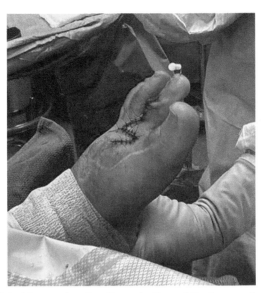

Fig. 31. Intraop clinical image showing the reduction of the hammertoe and final clinical image in the clinic.

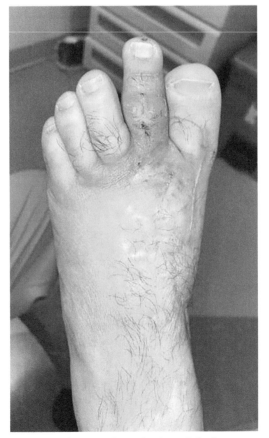

Fig. 32. Intraop clinical image showing the reduction of the hammertoe and final clinical image in the clinic.

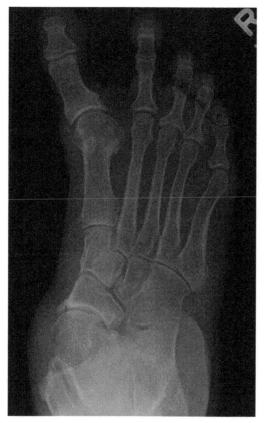

Fig. 33. Preop XRs demonstrating hallux varus and severe pes plano valgus foot.

CASE 5

46 year old male with PMH for hyperlipidemia had a traumatic accident over 10 years ago. He underwent multiple surgeries to save his foot and spent many days in the hospital to have local wound care and multiple rounds of antibiotics for osteomyelitis involving his first ray. He had a first MTPJ fusion due to the comminution associated with his fracture. He presented for second opinion for pain with his second digit hammertoe which was present but not addressed when they performed his first MTPJ fusion due to soft tissue healing issues (**Figs. 28–30**). After the discussion of options, it was elected to perform a Z-plasty at the second MTPJ level with arthrodesis of the second PIPJ with pinning and flexor tendon transfer. The preoperative discussion

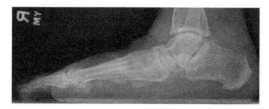

Fig. 34. Preop XRs demonstrating hallux varus and severe pes plano valgus foot.

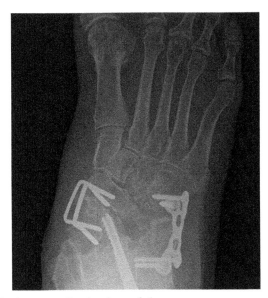

Fig. 35. Postop XRs demonstrating hardware failure.

with the patient addressed the potential healing issues since he had so much previous trauma, damage, and scar tissue formation from his original injury. He was amenable to the proposed plan, and the surgery went well. Fortunately, he had no skin healing issues, and he is currently walking without issues postoperatively (**Figs. 31** and **32**).

CASE 6

66-year-old female with osteoarthritis of multiple joints, chronic low back pain, and posterior tibial tendon dysfunction treated for many years with custom insoles, Richie brace, Arizona brace, and shoe modifications. She was sent to for second opinion for reconstruction. She had severe rearfoot arthritis with valgus position as well as a hallux varus without previous bunion surgery or known trauma to the toe (**Figs. 33** and **34**). For her first surgery, she underwent a gastrocnemius recession and triple arthrodesis, and it was elected to address her hallux varus at another date in the consideration of demand for skin healing. The patient was also hesitant to have the hallux varus fixed since it was not causing her pain currently. Interestingly enough, she had a skin reaction to the prep used during surgery, so for her first postoperative visit, she was given a boot to allow her to apply hydrocortisone cream to her lower leg. Although she was converted to a CAM boot, she was supposed to be non-weight bearing (**Figs. 35** and **36**).

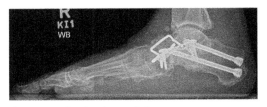

Fig. 36. Postop XRs demonstrating hardware failure.

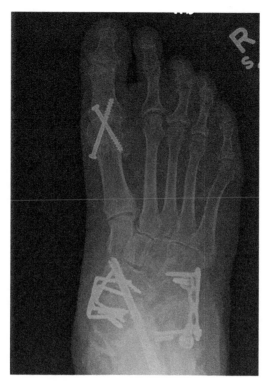

Fig. 37. Postop XRs from revision procedure.

At 4 weeks postoperatively, hardware failure (HWF) was identified. The patient had taken off her boot to walk around to the bathroom at home. A discussion was had about her being able to remain non-weight bearing to consider revision surgery, and if she could get extra assistance at home to help with household activities. She agreed that she able to meet all the needs discussed. For the revision surgery, more robust staples we in addition to bone graft material and the first MTPJ fusion was performed as well since the patient did not want to have a third surgery on this side. Betadine prep was used this surgery and she was kept in a cast postoperatively until 8 weeks postop. She healed well and is ambulating without issue on this side. She has ankle arthritis, but for now, her rearfoot fusion has allowed her to return to her activities and travel with her husband again (**Figs. 37** and **38**).

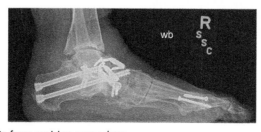

Fig. 38. Postop XRs from revision procedure.

SUMMARY

The key to success for any surgical misadventures is having honest conversations with your patients and figuring out what portion of the process contributed to the outcome. Sometimes this requires thinking outside of the box and sometimes it requires going back to the basics of bone healing and surgical technique. For these cases, almost all had pitfalls at multiple sections whether it was the patients' comorbidities, compliance, choice of surgery, and choice of fixation. The success for some of the patients relied heavily on medical management by their primary physicians. It is imperative to utilize other physicians for help with the management of our patients. Other cases relied on ensuring that the patient had the appropriate help at home for their recovery process. Extended periods of nonweight bearing is difficult for most individuals. Some of the cases had outcomes due to their own anatomy, while others were due to the index procedure choice and choice of fixation. Attention to all of these details and a systematic workup for patients is key for success. Working closely with your patients about their overall goals will typically result in a good outcome.

CLINICS CARE POINTS

- Define the problem and decipher what step of the process contributed to the outcome.
- Be aggressive with your approach when its appropriate.
- Sometimes you may need to think outside of the box.
- Be honest with your patient about their outcome and what is needed for their revision surgery to produce a better outcome.

DISCLOSURE

The author has nothing to disclose.

REFERENCES

1. Deodhar AK, Rana RE. Surgical physiology of wound healing: a review. J Postgrad Med 1997;43(2):52–6.
2. Cottrell JA, Turner JC, Arinzeh TL, et al. The biology of bone and ligament healing. Foot Ankle Clin 2016;21(4):739–61.
3. Gelfman Daniel. Good (medical) judgment comes from experience, and experience comes from (medical) misfortune. Am J Med 2020;133(12):1374–5.
4. Konstantinides NN, Lehmann S. The impact of nutrition on wound healing. Crit Care Nurse 1993;13:25.
5. Ishikawa SN, Murphy GA, Richardson EG. The effect of smoking on hindfoot fusions. Foot Ankle Int 2002;23:996–8.
6. Lynde MJ, Sautter T, Hamilton GA, Schuberth JM. Complications after open reduction and internal fixation of ankle fractures in the elderly. Foot Ankle Surg 2012;18(2):103–7.

Shaping the Next Generation of Foot and Ankle Surgeons

Podiatric Surgical Residency Education at Kaiser Permanente Northern California

Christy M. King, DPM, FACFAS[a,b,*], Cristian Neagu, DPM, FACFAS[c], Gray Williams, DPM, FACFAS[d]

KEYWORDS

- Academics/Didactics • Clinical education • Resident feedback • Resident research
- Resident wellness • Surgical education • Surgical olympics • Surgical skills

KEY POINTS

- Podiatric residency training should include a well-rounded experience in the management of all aspects of foot and ankle care, including surgery, clinical practice, academics, and research.
- Balanced surgical training is critical to produce successful podiatric surgeons. This experience should involve a variety of procedures, increasing degrees of autonomy, and supportive environment with more immediate feedback to assist the resident's growth.
- Clinical experiences are also essential to build a well-rounded clinician and can involve resident clinics where they are able to develop discussion skills with patients, work on evaluation techniques, and create treatment plans.
- The residents' clinical education should be augmented with various didactic sessions, including cadaver labs, simulation labs, saw bone workshops, journal club, resident lectures, attending lectures, and various other academics to strengthen their knowledge of the many aspects of foot and ankle pathology and treatment.

Continued

INTRODUCTION

Podiatric residency is only three short, yet comprehensive, years of a young resident's life where the goals are to gather as many opportunities and experiences in all facets of

[a] Department of Foot & Ankle Surgery, Kaiser Permanente, Oakland, CA, USA; [b] Kaiser San Francisco Bay Area Foot & Ankle Residency Program, Oakland, CA, USA; [c] Kaiser Santa Clara, 710 Lawrence Expressway Department 140, Santa Clara, CA 95051, USA; [d] Kaiser Vallejo, 975 Sereno Drive, Vallejo, CA 94589, USA
* Corresponding author. Department of Foot & Ankle Surgery, Kaiser Permanente, 275 Macarthur, Clinic 17, Oakland, CA 94611.
E-mail address: Christykingdpm@gmail.com

Clin Podiatr Med Surg 41 (2024) 193–210
https://doi.org/10.1016/j.cpm.2023.06.007
0891-8422/24/© 2023 Elsevier Inc. All rights reserved.

podiatric.theclinics.com

Continued

- Performing research in residency can increase knowledge, teach residents how to critically understand and discuss a certain topic, help build their accomplishments to assist in finding a job after residency, and reflect their expertise to patients.
- Developing a healthy work life balance is essential for leading a fulfilled and rewarding career and life. It is important to integrate the work team and family life to support the resident.

foot and ankle management to be prepared to handle any situation that they encounter as an individual practitioner in their career. The Council of Podiatric Medical Education (CPME) developed the CPME 320 document to present standards and requirements for all podiatric surgical residency programs.[1] There are hundreds of podiatric residency programs in the country, each helping to mold the future generation of podiatrists. While there are varying opinions on what truly makes a great residency program, the three separate Kaiser Permanente Northern California (KPNC) podiatric residency programs within the San Francisco (SF) Bay Area, which include Kaiser San Francisco Bay Area Foot & Ankle Residency Program (Oakland), Kaiser South Bay Consortium (Santa Clara), and Kaiser North Bay Consortium (Vallejo), strive to provide a comprehensive educational experience for our residents in a supportive and enjoyable environment.

The three KPNC podiatric residency programs operate independently out of separate regions of the San Francisco Bay Area, but work together to share experiences in all facets of education to optimize the opportunities for all of the KPNC podiatric residency programs (**Fig. 1**). The Kaiser San Francisco Bay Area Foot & Ankle Residency Program (Kaiser SF) rotates out of the center of the Bay Area in San Francisco, Oakland, and Diablo Service Area (Walnut Creek, Antioch, and Dublin). Kaiser South Bay Consortium (Kaiser SC) rotates out of Santa Clara and San Leandro. Kaiser North Bay Consortium (Kaiser NC) rotates out of Vallejo, San Rafael, and Santa Rosa. Working within each of these different communities helps to provide a diverse array of populations with a vast variety of pathologies.

HISTORY OF SURGICAL RESIDENCY PROGRAMS

The idea of formal surgical training programs was first introduced by Sir William Halstead in 1889 at Johns Hopkins University, and over the last 130 years, surgical residency training has expanded by leaps and bounds in all specialties, including podiatry.[2] Within KPNC, Hayward and Vallejo were the first locations to begin programs in the 1970's as podiatry itself was evolving within the system. It was quickly followed by Kaiser Oakland, who was one of the first to develop a 2-year and then a 3-year residency program. Even from the initial integration of podiatrists into the KPNC system, residency education was an essential part of podiatry's growth and development.

SURGICAL TRAINING

All podiatric residency programs seek to provide surgical and clinical training exposure to help mold competent and intelligent podiatric physicians and surgeons. Similar to the concept that it takes 10,000 hours of experience to become a master in the field of sports, this can also be applied to surgical residency training. The hope is that the more learning opportunities and mentorship provided in the surgical field, the closer

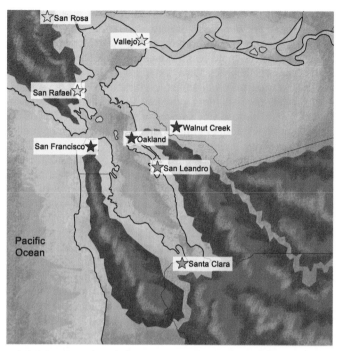

Fig. 1. Map of the San Francisco (SF) Bay Area and location of each of the podiatric residency programs. Kaiser San Francisco Bay Area Foot & Ankle Residency Program rotates out of the center of the SF Bay Area in San Francisco, Oakland, and Walnut Creek area (blue stars). Kaiser South Bay Consortium rotates out of Santa Clara and San Leandro (green stars). Kaiser North Bay Consortium rotates out of Vallejo, San Rafael, and Santa Rosa (yellow stars).

our residents can become experts in the field of foot and ankle surgery. To assist in defining the minimum experiences required, the CPME 320 developed standards requirements for case and procedure activities (**Table 1**).[2] Within KPNC podiatric residency program locations, the podiatric surgeons perform almost all, if not all, of the

Table 1
CPME 320 requirements as of July 1st, 2023

Procedural Activities	Required Cases	Example of Kaiser Resident Case Numbers above required
First and second assistant procedures (total)	400	4x
Digital	80	2x
First Ray	60	4x
Other Soft Tissue Foot Surgery	45	5x
Other Osseous Foot Surgery	40	4x
Reconstructive Rearfoot/Ankle (added credential only)	50	8x

care for the foot and ankle, including trauma, reconstruction, total ankle replacements, arthroscopy, forefoot surgery, midfoot surgery, and rearfoot surgery (**Fig. 2**).

Unlike medicine-based training programs where the majority of education is provided in the form of didactic lectures and patient interactions, in surgical programs the exposure to core surgical procedures and more importantly the "hands on" interaction is crucial. Literature from general surgery training programs have discussed important factors in this process. First, *operative experience* which in a sense corresponds to availability and exposure to surgical cases.[3] Within the KPNC podiatric residency programs, surgical volumes at graduations have historically been more than double if not even more than the assigned minimum activity volume (MAV) for graduation (see **Table 1**). Most residents will graduate with more than 1000 cases. Also, it is important to appreciate the difference between procedures performed versus cases as they are counted for podiatric surgical training. Each patient with their associated procedures will count as one case. However, a bunionectomy with hammertoe procedures on the 2nd and 3rd would count as three procedures while a flat foot reconstruction may only count as one procedure. Evaluating both the quality and quantity of procedures and cases is essential to understand the experiences a program can provide. The second factor is *operative teaching* aimed at providing the resident with progressive autonomy as they progress through their residency. This in turn leads to an increase in resident engagement and motivation. In this process the leadership and experience of the faculty is paramount. Aside from being active at the national and international level teaching at professional meetings, KPNC podiatric surgeons have been able to routinely address not only the basic anatomic approaches and pathology but also advanced topics such as preoperative planning, surgical approaches, and management of complications.

CLINICAL TRAINING

While residency training may seem to focus on podiatric surgical training, providing experiences in various clinics is essential to training a well-rounded podiatric clinician. Each of the KPNC podiatric residency program sites have various opportunities including preoperative clinic, post operative clinic, trauma clinic, podopediatric clinic, wound care clinic, ingrown toenail clinic, complicated reconstruction consultation clinic, and special problems group clinic to name a few. There is a dearth of literature to support how much clinical experiences are recommended for graduating residents. The previous CPME 320 guidelines recommended 1000 clinic encounters while the new CPME 320 guidelines recommend at least 100 procedures which can include

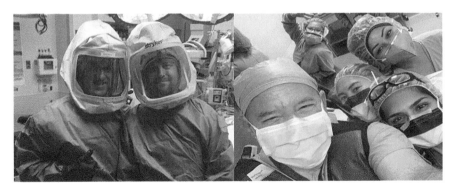

Fig. 2. Building resident and attending relationships in the operating room.

nail avulsions or matricectomies, ankle reductions, and injections to highlight a few. At some sites, residents assist attendings with the clinic while other sites have more specific resident run clinics. Some of this variation is due to department needs along with ensuring appropriate resident supervision, patient communication, and follow up. A study by Bischoff and colleagues surveyed podiatric residents about resident run clinics and found 59.79% of the residents interviewed had a resident run clinic and 89.66% of those residents liked having a resident run clinic.[4] Opinions may differ as to the ideal type and amount of clinical education; however, it is important to provide residents the opportunity to develop skills in the evaluation and formation of treatment plans for their patients.

DIDACTIC TRAINING

Incoming PGY-1 residents will invariably graduate from different medical schools with different educational experiences, and it is fair to assume that their knowledge base will vary. It is therefore imperative for the residency program to have in place an academic schedule which takes into account the PGY training level of the resident and the complexity of pathology. The didactic portion of their education helps to augment the clinical and surgical hands-on experience the residents receive. While the CPME 320 dictates that journal club is required monthly, the remaining academic opportunities can be variable among programs and include, surgical labs, attending lectures, resident lectures, board review, and many more (**Fig. 3**). One of the advantages of practicing within the KPNC system is the existing strong regional and local Gradual Medical Education (GME) support, as well as, individual program autonomy. Within the three KPNC podiatric residency programs, we have worked to provide many different types of didactic activities beyond their direct patient care experiences. Each program has developed an extensive academic schedule to cover the important foot and ankle topics over the 3 years of training (**Table 2**).

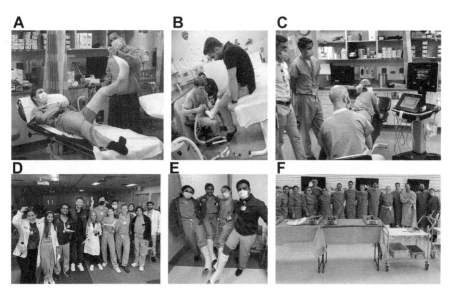

Fig. 3. Clinical and Surgical skills labs. (*A*) Ankle fracture reduction demonstration, (*B*) Casting workshop, (*C*) Ultrasound utilization, (*D*) Saw bones workshop, (*E*) Splint workshop, (*F*) Surgical cadaver lab.

Table 2
Example of 3-year schedule to capture important foot and ankle topics during a resident's three year career

Year 1	Topics
July	Orientation
August	General skills (surgical anatomy, incision approaches, operating room set up, common procedural techniques, external fixation, and so forth)
September	Cartilage science and pathology/Talar dome lesions
October	Ankle fractures management (including diabetic and geriatric)
November	Diabetes Mellitus: Medicine and Trauma
December	DVT/PVD prophylaxis and treatment (Vascular)
January	Orthoplastics/Dermatologic conditions
February	General Orthopedic Trauma and Emergencies
March	Calcaneal Fractures
April	First ray pathology (hallux valgus/hallux rigidus)
May	Tendon transfers utilization
June	Lesser ray pathology (MTPJ instability, digital and metatarsal deformity)
Year 2	**Topics**
July	Orientation
August	General skills (surgical anatomy, incision approaches, operating room set up, common procedural techniques, external fixation, and so forth)
September	Podiatric trauma and emergencies (soft tissue trauma, open fractures, compartment syndrome)
October	Ankle arthritis (arthrodesis and total ankle replacement)
November	Bone and soft tissue tumors
December	Anesthesia/Pain Management
January	Septic arthritis; Sero negative disorders/Rheumatoid Arthritis/Gout
February	Charcot arthropathy treatment and reconstruction
March	Congenital deformity (Clubfoot, metatarsus adductus, polydactyl, macrodactyly)
April	Talus fractures
May	Midfoot fractures (lisfrancs, navicular, cuboid)
June	Peroneal tendinopathy/lateral ankle instability
Year 3	**Topics**
July	Orientation
August	General skills (surgical anatomy, incision approaches, operating room set up, common procedural techniques, external fixation, and so forth)
September	Arthroscopy (Ankle, subtalar, and more)
October	Pilon fractures
November	Osteomyelitis/Infectious disease
December	Practice management/Occupational medicine/Medical legal
January	Bone science/fracture healing/nonunion/orthobiologics
February	Achilles ruptures and tendinopathy
March	Diabetic wound care and amputations/Limb salvage
April	Pes planus (adult and pediatric)
May	Neurologic disorders and treatment/Pes Cavus
June	Pediatric Fractures

The schedule rotates each year so that over their 3 years of training, they will receive didactic teaching in every subject.

Each residency program can tailor their curriculum to best fit the needs and personality of the program and residents. At Kaiser SC and Kaiser NC, protected educational time has been set aside one afternoon a week where attending lectures and hands on labs take place with the resident on site. At the Kaiser SF program, various additional educational conferences such as radiology rounds occur at lunch time a day per week with evening academics once a week where all residents join together. In addition, M&M and monthly attending lectures also take place in which attendings and residents clinical time is held to share in the didactic education.

Didactic Training: Academics

The academic portion of resident education can involve many different training modules. Journal club is required monthly and helps the residents to learn to critically read and interpret the literature. To assist the resident in their evaluation of the monthly journal club articles and leading the discussion, we developed a concise set of questions for each resident to present their selected article (**Fig. 4**). Attending lectures can be a valuable addition as there are many experienced foot and ankle attendings within our programs that also lecture on a national scale, and our residents are able to learn from them on a daily basis. With relationships our attendings have developed across the country and even internationally, we have been able to have various visiting attendings present on their unique practice (**Fig. 5**). Utilizing unique approaches to education, a Jeopardy-based game discussing important foot and ankle topics, can help present questions important for board testing and solidify their knowledge while doing it in entertaining manner (**Fig. 6**). Multiple other skills are included in training such as casting workshops and ultrasound utilization (**Fig. 3**). Resident lectures help the resident critically organize their understanding of common foot and ankle conditions as well as strengthen their presentation skills. In the post-pandemic world, both in-person and virtual academics has been utilized to balance academic commitments and resident wellness. There are so many ways to augment the residents' education and using a well-rounded approach to their didactic education supports their grasp of various subjects in foot and ankle knowledge.

Journal Club Article Evaluation Tool

Title

Purpose + Hypothesis: Should be clearly stated in the last 2 sentences of the paper's introduction

Methods: How did they organize their study. Include type of study, n, and what they did including primary and secondary aims.

Significant results: What were the significant results? (Only need to share significant results OR things that were interestingly not significant. In other words, you don't have to discuss every result)

What are the strengths and weakness of the research?

How does this change or augment your practice (Think if this would change your practice now or after residency), How and/or why (or why not)

What are the next research steps to explore this subject?

How can this study be expanded upon to further the literature base?

Fig. 4. Journal Club Evaluation tool helps to lead an educational and concise academic session.

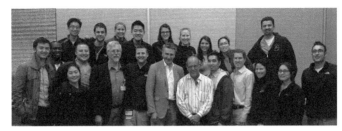

Fig. 5. Visiting faculty, orthopedic traumatology surgeon from Germany, Dr. Krettek.

Didactic Training: Surgical Labs

When building confidence in surgical skills, it is important to practice the procedures in a controlled environment with either simulators, saw bones, and cadaver labs. The main advantage of cadaver labs aside from accurate anatomic representation is lack of time constraints and external pressures.[5] In addition, accurate representation of pathology and hands on learning has been shown to reduce medical errors and increase patient safety.[6] In a study by Chu and colleagues, they explored the effectiveness of cadaver labs in podiatric residency training. Of the 173 podiatric residents who responded to the survey, representing 74 residency programs, 87.9% of the respondents felt that a cadaver lab was extremely (57.8%) or somewhat beneficial (30.1%).[5] Similar to the national trend where the majority of cadaver labs are industry sponsored, KPNC residents are able to have access to instrumentation from multiple vendors vetted by the Kaiser Permanente system. This provides not only exposure to hardware employed for all facets of foot and ankle surgery but also to faculty members who are routinely involved in nationally sponsored resident training courses. Surgical hands-on labs can help to increase resident knowledge and comfort with procedural steps and increase their appreciation of anatomy and planes of dissection. Surgical skills labs at each program have included arthroscopy labs (**Fig. 7**), saw bone, and external fixator workshops to name a few (**Fig. 8**). While surgical training labs may not eliminate possible complications during an actual procedure, they serve as another avenue to improve surgical skills and build confidence in a procedure.

Didactic Training: Surgical Olympics

Surgical Olympics have been integrated into various programs around the country in different medical fields to further augment the surgical education in a fun yet increased spirited environment. Within the Kaiser SF Bay Area program, the residents are on teams of three with a PGY-1, PGY-2, and PGY-3 on each team. Throughout the year, the residents compete with their teams in various academics such as hands on labs, jeopardy, board review, and other academics to build points for their team

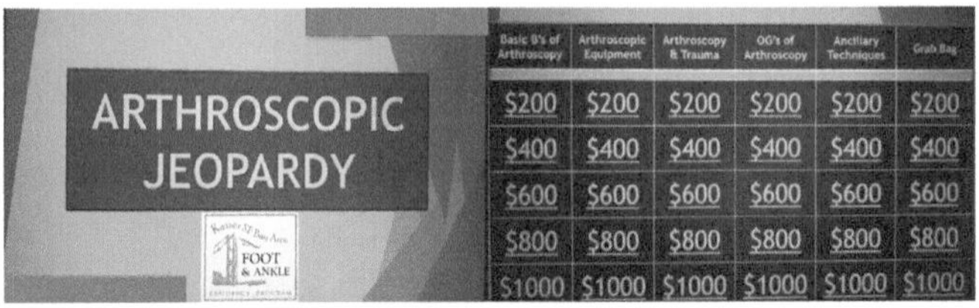

Fig. 6. An example of arthroscopy Jeopardy for weekly academics.

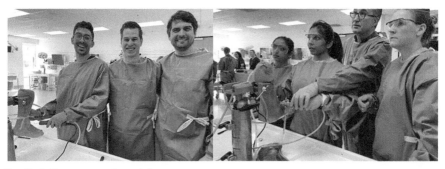

Fig. 7. Arthroscopy cadaver labs.

for the final surgical olympics competition at the end of the academic year in June. At the end of year surgical competition, the residents perform tasks deemed appropriate for their level of training for their team in a timed environment, and the winning team is crowned (**Figs. 9** and **10**). A study by Oberoi and colleagues explored how a surgical skills Olympiad in a general surgery residency improved resident performance, and they found that over 90% of the evaluators noted that the Olympiad was beneficial for the residents and helped to assess their skills.[7] More important that declaring a winner, all of the residents benefit from a enjoyable and challenging situation to hone their dexterity and understanding of common podiatric principles and skills.

RESEARCH

Attempting to complete research during a busy surgical residency training program can sometimes feel such as a daunting task; however, it can be a very rewarding experience not only to increase ones' own knowledge of a topic within foot and ankle, but also helps to progress the profession, support a resident's expertise when they are

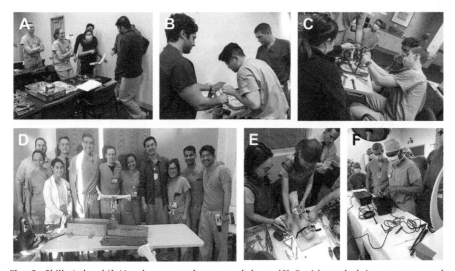

Fig. 8. Skills Labs. (*A*) Hands on saw bone workshop, (*B*) Residents helping mentor each other, (*C*) External fixation lab, (*D*) Ankle fracture saw bones workshop, (*E*) Total ankle workshop, (*F*) Arthroscopic simulation.

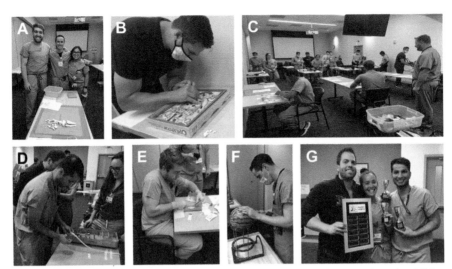

Fig. 9. Surgical olympics. (*A*) 2020 winning team, (*B*) Resident working on dexterity, (*C*) Surgical Olympics room setup, (*D*) Working on Achilles tendon Krakow technique, (*E*) PGY1 Olympic skill; suturing, (*F*) Keeping the external fixation wires parallel to the fixation bar through a simulated leg (watermelon), (*G*) Inagural winning team.

looking for jobs or applying for privileges, and even help with a patient's confidence in a provider. The KPNC system prides itself on assisting in research in multiple areas of the medical profession and has supportive departments, such as the Division of Research (DOR) and the Institutional Review Board (IRB), that assist residents and their attending principle investigators to complete high-quality research within their three years of training. In addition to experienced and enthusiastic attendings to contribute to the research, there is also local assistance from research coordinators at each residency program to aid the residents in IRB protocol formation, research methodology training, manuscript creation, and presentations. The residents are able to take their completed research manuscripts and posters to national conferences to further their abilities to present and develop connections across the country (**Fig. 11**).

RESEARCH: KAISER FOOT AND ANKLE RESIDENCY RESEARCH SUMMIT

Every spring, the three KPNC podiatric residency programs join to celebrate both resident and student research at the Kaiser Permanente Foot & Ankle Residency Research Summit (**Fig. 12**). At the event, Kaiser residents present their completed

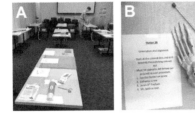
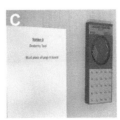
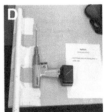

Fig. 10. Examples of surgical Olympic stations. (*A*) Surgical Olympics room set up, (*B*) Orienting hardware, (*C*) Dexterity tool, (*D*) Drill without plunging.

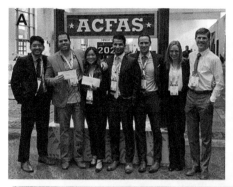
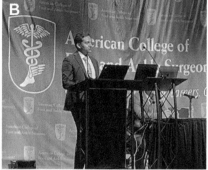
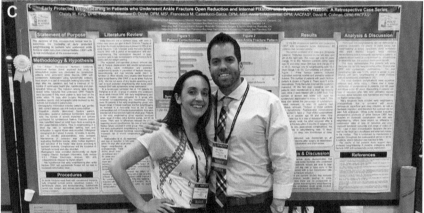

Fig. 11. Resident Research. (*A*) Manuscript and poster presenters at ACFAS, (*B*) Resident presenting his research at the manuscript presentation track at national conference, (*C*) Residents awarded for poster research.

or ongoing research to their peers and attendings from around the San Francisco Bay Area. In addition, students from all of the podiatry schools are invited to submit an abstract of their research, and some are selected for a travel stipend supported by our Kaiser Regional GME department to present their poster at the event. The event helps to build connections across the region and allows the residents to present their research in a supportive environment to strengthen their presentation skills and the research project itself prior to formal presentation at a conference.

Wellness

Even before the pandemic, medical professionals were struggling to find a balance between all of their work responsibilities, taking quality care of their patients, and investing in their own personal health and family wellness. With the COVID pandemic and extra weight placed on the shoulders of medicine, it became essential to invest in the wellbeing of our medical professionals, including our residents. Residency will be a more challenging part of anyone's career; however, it is important to find a supportive environment that can maximize both your education and personal wellness.

Resident wellness over the last few years has become a very important topic in the process of training a young physician. Aside from achieving a better quality of life via work-life balance, resident wellness is closely associated with the ability of residents

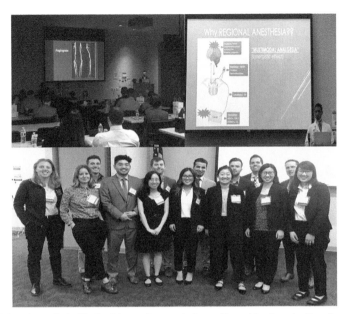

Fig. 12. Kaiser Foot & Ankle Residency Research Summit, resident and attending presentations along with photo of resident presenters from all three KPNC podiatric residency programs.

to complete their surgical training programs. Despite the fact that little data is available on this topic in the podiatric surgical residency programs, multiple articles have documented this process in general surgery residency training. Sullivan and colleagues looked at 2,033 categorical PGY-1 and PGY-2 residents and found that concerns regarding personal sacrifice required, less than ideal relationship with faculty and peers, length of surgical training, and day-to-day experience to be important factors contributing to attrition.[8]

The process of identifying risk factors for residents in the attrition group is complex. Studies focused on single institutions may provide clear data, however, they do not take into consideration geographic location and size of the programs which have also been found to be important factors. Kelz and coworkers found that male sex was independently protective against attrition in a group of 600 general surgery residents.[9] This finding was mirrored by separate studies by Aufses and Bergen who found that the rate of attrition in women was 2.2 times higher than that of men.[10,11] These results may highlight how traditional residency training was constructed more for the male gender, however, it is critical to find resources and mentorship within the residency program to support the female residency training experience as well. Within the KPNC programs, mentorship groups have been developed to assist in strengthening the resident experience for all. Other studies however have contested the gender discrepancy, and have instead, found attrition rates to be closely associated with age greater than 29 and academic and extracurricular variables.[12] Yeo and associates in their multivariate analysis identified PGY-1 status as the only demographic factor associated with attrition.[13] This finding along with program location and multiple resident attitudes were also identified as independent resident attrition factors in Sullivan's study. Interestingly, the 20% attrition rate was not found to be associated with program size, working conditions, or sex composition of the resident group.

Resident attrition within the KPNC podiatric programs is negligible. The highly competitive, yet supportive, nature of the residencies attracts not only the brightest of students but also students with a drive to learn and a strong work ethic. In addition to a very well balanced and organized academic schedule, the emphasis on resident well-being has led to very good education and life balance, an important factor for the new generation of residents and residency training.

In addition to focusing on resident wellness, mentorship has been shown to be an important factor in the advancement of young physician careers.[14] A mentor can provide advice, guidance, professional personal support which has been shown to lead to successful and fruitful careers as well as enhance personal happiness.[15] At the KPNC podiatric residency programs, incoming PGY-1 residents are assigned a mentor based on their personality, interests, and goals. This relationship is based on mutual respect and has been crucial in helping the young physicians make the transition from medical school to surgical residency.

WELLNESS: RESIDENT RETREAT

To assist in building resident relationships and the family environment, residents are encouraged to create a resident retreat event annually where an attending takes primary call, so that the residents are able to take full advantage of their time together without the worry of interruption from the pager (**Fig. 13**). In the past, residents have organized events such as dinners, hiking trips, Napa Valley wine tours, golfing adventures, and other activities to spend time together in various amazing regions of the San Francisco Bay Area.

WELLNESS: ATTENDING AND RESIDENT WELLNESS EVENTS

Resident and attendings enjoy interactions with each other outside of the work environment to help share experiences and strengthen relationships. Wellness events have included attendings versus resident sports events such as basketball, kickball, bowling, mini golf, and go cart racing (**Fig. 14**). Family responsibilities and the work team can sometimes be considered competing interests; however, it is essential to integrate the traditional family and work family whenever possible to further solidify the resident support system (**Fig. 15**). The KPNC podiatric residency programs take advantage of finding time to spend together whenever possible.

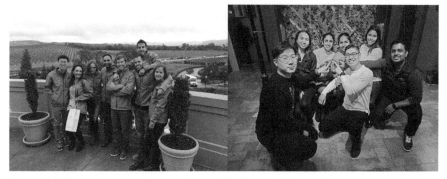

Fig. 13. Residency Retreat to Napa Valley while the attending holds the pager.

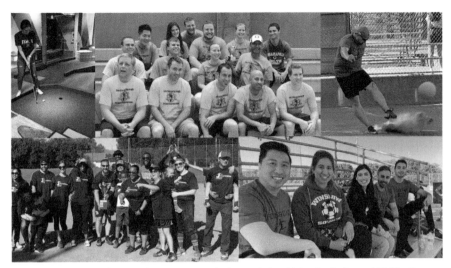

Fig. 14. Resident and Attending events including mini golf, basketball, and kickball

ADDITIONAL EDUCATIONAL EXPERIENCES: MISSION TRIPS AND FELLOWSHIP OPPORTUNITIES

While not required for surgical training, there are supplementary opportunities that can not only further surgical and clinical knowledge and skills, but also ultimately open our eyes to the vast experiences of others around the world. This can come in forms of volunteering locally like with the special Olympics, traveling on medical mission trips, or completeing mini fellowships. With the support of KPNC, residents and attendings

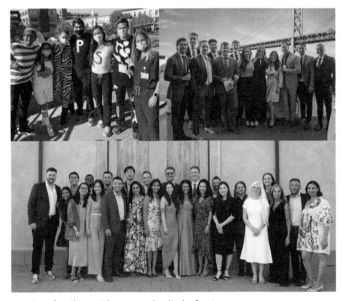

Fig. 15. Integrating family, residency, and a little fun!.

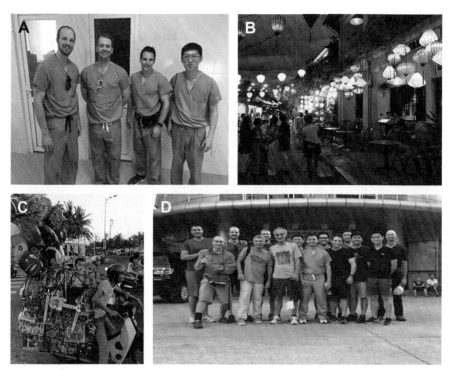

Fig. 16. Da Nang, Vietnam Mission trip. (*A*) Resident attendees, (*B*) Local experiences, (*C*) Street vendor, (*D*) Attending and resident team.

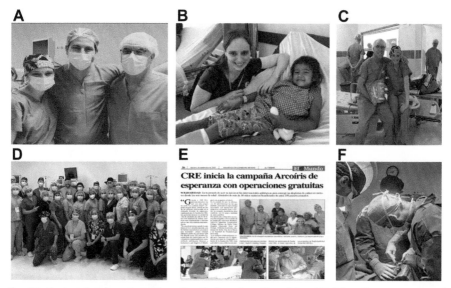

Fig. 17. Project Rainbow to various South American Countries. (*A*) Attending surgeon and resident attendees, (*B*) Chief resident Dr Tenaya West with patient, (*C*) Dr. Silvani and Dr. West getting ready for the day, (*D*) Bolivia mission team, (*E*) Local newspaper covers Project Rainbow's visit, (*F*) Attending and Resident in Surgery. Photos A-C took place in Boliva 2019, provided courtesy Dr Tenaya West. Photos D-F took place in Bolivia 2022, courtesy of Dr. Joseph Dickinson.

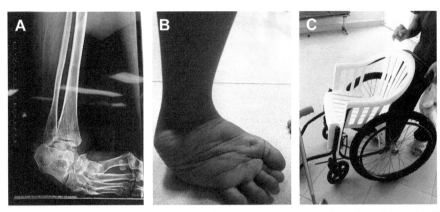

Fig. 18. Example of deformity encountered on Da Nang mission trip. (*A*) Radiograph, (*B*) Clinical photos, (*C*) Wheelchair used for the mission trip. (Photos courtesy of Dr. Gray Williams.)

are able to donate their time to local communities or travel to various mission trips around the world. The most common mission trips attended include either Da Nang in Vietnam (**Fig. 16**) or Project Rainbow that helps various communities throughout South America (**Fig. 17**). At each of these medical missions, residents are exposed to complex neglected foot and ankle conditions (**Figs. 18** and **19**). These experiences are incredibly rewarding in so many ways. In addition, our residents have had the opportunity to pursue a mini fellowship in Switzerland with world renowned orthopedic surgeon, Dr Klaue, where they are able to see diverse ways to treat foot and ankle deformity and trauma. These diverse experiences help to build a well rounded clinician and surgeon.

Providing resident feedback

Providing feedback is an important part of residency training to help the identify areas of improvement. The so-called "feedback sandwich" has been proposed as a way to give effective feedback by starting and ending with encouraging words with the constructive feedback in between. This may be a good way to start the feedback conversation after you observe errors or the need for improvement, but it does run the risk of being formulaic. A more effective three-pronged approach has been developed for

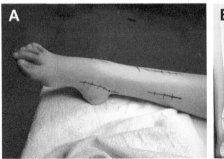
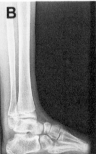
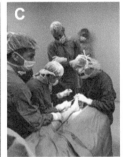

Fig. 19. (*A*) Clinical images of deformity encountered on previous Da Nang mission trips, (*B*) Radiographs, (*C*) Attending and residents performing surgery.

teaching procedural skills but can be extrapolated to most teaching opportunities. This method follows the pattern of 1) Prebrief, 2) During Procedure, and 3) Debrief. With this more proactive model, surgical resident teaching is more intentional and incorporates the resident in the process of evaluating, critiquing, and improving their performance.

- *Prebrief*: The resident and faculty discuss possible challenges that may present during the procedure. This is a great opportunity for the faculty to convey what they are planning, any challenges specific to the case, and assess the resident's level of preparedness.
- *During the procedure*: The teaching faculty can focus on what was discussed and provide guidance directed at the issues in question or ask cogent questions.
- *Debrief*: The resident is provided with time to reflect on their performance. At this point, faculty initiate a discussion of what the resident thinks went well or could have gone better then discuss specific skills to focus on and ways to improve in the future.

SUMMARY

To further deliver our profession to the pinnacle, it is paramount that we invest in all aspects of our podiatric residency training to help mentor the next generation of foot and ankle clinicians and surgeons. From very early on in the acceptance and integration of podiatry into the KPNC model, podiatric residency training been an essential part of many KPNC podiatry departments. Not only are the attendings extremely committed to teaching, but also the GME department supports the podiatric residents with great respect and parity. The three KPNC residency programs are proud to provide comprehensive experiences in all aspects of podiatric training and look forward to seeing our residents and the profession reach great heights.

CLINICS CARE POINTS

- Podiatric Residency is three short years to gain as much experience with all aspect of foot and ankle pathology and treatment to set up the resident for a successful and fufilling career on graduation.
- It is important to find a residency training program with a comprehensive surgical training with large quantity of cases, extensive case quality, and mentorship to augment the education.
- Clinical evaluation and treatment is essential to experience to prepare for the post-residency career.
- Utilizing various approaches to academic education further expands the residents' knowledge and hands-on skills.
- Research performed during residency training can further add to the resident's instruction.
- Residency training will be a demanding time in anyone's career. Finding a program that provides a well balanced education along with mentorship and healthy work-life balance is essential.

DISCLOSURE

The authors have nothing to disclose.

REFERENCES

1. Standards and requirements for approval of podiatric medicine and surgery residencies. 2023 https://www.cpme.org/files
2. Cameron JL. William Stewart Halsted. Our surgical heritage, Ann Surg, 1997;225(5):445–458.
3. Abbott KL, Krumm AE, Kelley JK, et al. Society for Improving Medical Professional Learning. Surgical Trainee Performance and Alignment With Surgical Program Director Expectations. Ann Surg 2022;276(6). e1095-e1100.
4. Bischoff AJ, Stone R, Dao T, et al. The resident-run clinic in podiatric medical foot and ankle surgery residency training: a study of resident-perceived benefit. J Am Podiatr Med Assoc 2022;112(6):21–152.
5. Chu AK, Law RW, Greschner JM, et al. Effectiveness of the cadaver lab in podiatric surgery residency programs. J Foot Ankle Surg 2020;59(2):246–52.
6. Holland JP, Waugh L, Horgan A, et al. Cadaveric hands-on training for surgical specialties: is this back to the future for surgical skills development? J Surg Educ 2011;68:110–6.
7. Oberoi KPS, Caine AD, Schwartzman J, et al. Surgical skills Olympiad: a 4-year experience in a general surgery residency program. Surg J 2021;7(3):e222–5.
8. Sullivan MC, Yeo H, Roman S, et al. Surgical residency and attrition:defining the individual and programmatic factors predictive of trainee loss. J Am Coll Surg 2013;216(3):461–71.
9. Kelz RR, Mullen JL, Kaiser LR, et al. Prevention of surgical resident attrition by a novel selection strategy. Ann Surg 2010;252:537e541 [discussion: 541e533].
10. Aufses AH, Slater GI, Hollier LH. The nature and fate of categorical surgical residents who "drop out". Am J Surg 1998;175:236e239.
11. Bergen PC, Turnage RH, Carrico CJ. Gender-related attrition in a general surgery training program. J Surg Res 1998;77:59e62.
12. Naylor RA, Reisch JS, Valentine RJ. Factors related to attrition in surgery residency based on application data. Arch Surg 2008;143:647e651 [discussion: 651e652].
13. Yeo H, Bucholz E, Ann Sosa J, et al. A national study of attrition in general surgery training: which residents leave and where do they go? Ann Surg 2010;252:529e534 [discussion: 534e526].
14. Reghunathan M, Crowley J, Gosman A. Plastic surgery diversity, equity, and inclusion mentorship program and workshop: a single institution's experience. Plast Reconstr Surg 2023;151(1):227.
15. Rohrich R, Durand P. Mentors, leaders, and role models: Same or different? Plast Reconstr Surg 2020;145(4):1099–101.

Epilogue: One Job

John M. Schuberth, DPM[a,b,*]

KEYWORDS

• Career • Retirement • Podiatric medicine • Foot and ankle surgery

As I reflect on almost 40 years of clinical practice, it dawned on me that I have really only held one job in my professional career (**Figs. 1** and **2**). I remember the first day like it was yesterday, and I remember the last day, but the in between represents my soul, a soul that has been shaped by countless experiences. Some of these experiences were immediately impactful and left an indelible mark on my soul, but most of them were memorable only for a fleeting moment, soon to be forgotten. Yet the cumulation of these seemingly trivial experiences, in retrospect, served as the foundation of my career at Kaiser Permanente.

I would often get annoyed when patients or colleagues would refer to Kaiser as if it was a person. Frequently, in jest, I would ask for Kaiser's first or last name, only to be met with a blank stare. However, the personification of this particular health plan is not entirely obtuse. As a provider and consumer of health care, it became clear to me that any patient's experience is mostly shaped by the people connected to that event. Whether it be a physician, surgeon, nurse, radiology technician, receptionist, or medical assistant, these are all people, Human interaction cannot be avoided or ignored but I have learned that as a provider, my ability to provide care that was consistent with my values and pursuit of perfection, depended largely on my ability and commitment to motivate other people. I have fond memories of a radiology technician that was often assigned to my operating room (OR) during ankle replacements. Early on, he struggled to keep up with me, and I became increasingly frustrated. Finally, I called his supervisor and asked if I could train him. I took him into the OR on my own time, with a C-arm, and demonstrated what was expected. Over time, he became one of the best technicians I have ever experienced. He was so grateful that when *he* retired, he gave *me* a present.

I learned that those that we work with are indeed "people" that have lives outside of the workplace and these interests occasionally collided, much like mine did. As such, in my position as a surgeon, or any surgeon, there is an implied obligation to be a leader. I learned that the captain of the ship doctrine does not necessarily hold true if the shipmates are planning a mutiny. A mutiny not in the historical sense where the captain is tossed overboard, but a mutiny staged primarily by indifference, passive

[a] Department of Orthopaedic Surgery, Foot and Ankle Surgery, Kaiser Permanente Medical Center, San Francisco, CA, USA; [b] Kaiser Foundation Hospital, 450 6th Avenue, San Francisco, CA 94118, USA
* Corresponding author.
E-mail address: jmfoot@aol.com

Clin Podiatr Med Surg 41 (2024) 211–214
https://doi.org/10.1016/j.cpm.2023.06.008
0891-8422/24/© 2023 Elsevier Inc. All rights reserved.

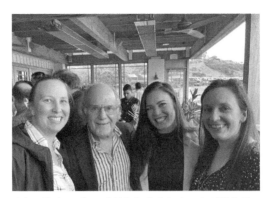

Fig. 1. From left to right, Christy King, DPM, Jack Schuberth, DPM, Shontal Dionisiopoulos, DPM, and Francesca Castellucci-Garza, DPM.

aggressiveness, and other counterproductive mannerisms. Accordingly, I tried to act in a fashion that fostered enthusiasm to be in my room. As a member of the executive committee of the OR, I was the conduit of complaints from the nursing and surgical technician staff about "certain surgeons." I did not want to be one of "those surgeons." Through humor and mutual respect, collectively, we had mostly good days in the OR. One of my colleagues had difficulty understanding why I always seemed to get an OR when I needed one. Perhaps it is because I did not pound my fist on the desk and verbally assault the charge nurse!

I learned that human resources is not a pleasurable destination. Obviously, it is a necessary component of large organizations, but it is not designed to solve issues, only to formally identify and document them. I realized that speaking your mind in a forthright fashion is a free and renewable ticket to human resources. I learned that once you are committed, it is not about right and wrong, it is about protection of the organization. "One and done" became my mantra after the initial episode. Not surprisingly, my opinions never changed. I just kept them to myself!

I learned that if patients trust you, they will ride out complications with you. In the modern era, that trust is not axiomatic to the initial stages of the doctor-patient relationship. You have to earn it, and then keep it throughout the journey. The best way

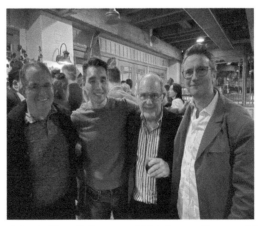

Fig. 2. From left to right, Jeffrey Christensen, DPM, Danny Choung, DPM, Jack Schuberth, DPM, and Lawrence Ford, DPM.

to earn trust is to be humble. Although humility is not frequently associated with any surgeon, it goes a long way. A blend of humility, confidence, honesty, and reputation establish the framework of a solid doctor-patient relationship, even when things do not go as planned. I think it is hard to understand this concept early in one's career simply because most of us have not yet been on the other side of the knife. I have had 11 operations (9 of them orthopedic) and aside from the three minor hand surgeries, I was notably scared. I also learned how to be a better doctor by letting someone else doctor me. After my rotator cuff surgery, synovial fluid kept draining from the portal 5 weeks postoperative. I had carefully chosen this highly experienced orthopedist, who had done more than 1000 cuff repairs. He kept reassuring me that it would get better, even though I was convinced I would need another operation to close it. Mind you, even though I had scant knowledge of shoulder surgery, I did not get on Google, nor challenge him, because I trusted him. Had I needed another procedure, I wanted him to do it. Turns out he was right, and I was able to regain full function of my shoulder in short order.

I learned that every single patient deserves the same treatment you would want for yourself or your family. Every single patient deserves the same care regardless of their socioeconomic status, political persuasions, or any of the other differentiating characteristics that we assign to humanity. Perhaps it is not as easy as it seems, but this notion should never be discarded.

Not every patient needs an operation. Many patients get better without us. I remember a quote (although not the author) that states: "A good surgeon knows HOW to operate; a great surgeon knows WHEN to operate; but the best surgeon knows when NOT to operate." Honoring this tenet does not come with your diploma. Unfortunately, it comes only with a blend of experience and common sense. In residency the primary focus is learning foot and ankle surgery. We graduate, seeing mainly those patients that had operations. What we often lack is the experience of the process. We do not see interactions between surgeon and patient that culminate in a surgical case. I could not count the number of frustrating patient encounters revolving around a mismatch of patient and surgeon expectations. In most instances the surgery was done appropriately, but it was a surgery that may not have been necessary. Yes, the radiograph looked perfect, but did it really help the patient? I always wanted to pick up the telephone and ask, "Would you do the same thing if that patient was part of your family"? I never did because I already knew the answer.

Above all, I learned to be honest with patients. I learned how to have those difficult conversations, without any formal training whatsoever. It became easier and easier when I realized that all you need to do is tell people the truth. It is easier to tell them what you think they want to hear, or something that will deflect blame, but then you have to remember what you told them at the next encounter. You never have to recall the truth.

For years I have threatened to write a book about these and many more experiences during my professional career. I always thought it would be somewhat autobiographical, modeled after the humor and satire in the "The House of God." But I would not do it if I could not be more evocative, more emotional, and rawer. Although I think it is sorely needed, after retirement, the last thing I wanted was another job. One job was enough, and I would not have traded it with anyone.

Speaking of retirement, it has now been 100 days after my last one-man parade out of the OR. Needless to say, it was not easy, because I realized that I would never pitch my blood-soaked gloves into that ubiquitous red bin. Many have suggested and perhaps even covertly waged some money that I would be back at work in short order. In fact, I have been offered several opportunities to do just that. Yet, those that tried to predict my future presumably based their beliefs on my passion to take care of people. Conversely, I never thought about professional life after Kaiser. Somehow, I knew that this was the end. But that notion was not engraved on my soul until one seminal moment, a moment that in retrospect, I should have captured on my own many years ago. I was exchanging emails with a prominent orthopedic foot and ankle surgeon, after I was informed that he retired at the age of 60, clearly at the peak of his career. He had patients coming from all over the United States (and maybe even from abroad), to fix their total ankle miseries. I asked him what was going to happen to all of these patients now that he was retired. He told me that he retired because if he kept going, one of these days someone else was going to make the decision and that someone else would be his health. In essence, he said that no one can do this forever and the only definitive is that there will be an end. Once I digested the reality, it was remarkably easy to pull the trigger. However, the pathway to the end was tortuous! Once I had casted a retirement date 9 to 12 months henceforth, I began to tell patients and colleagues of the impending hiatus. Some scoffed, almost as if I was trying to garner some attention. Admittedly, I privately wondered whether they were right. Clarity arrived while I was on vacation with my family in the South African wine country. Two days before our scheduled return home, I developed severe abdominal pain, such that I could not eat or even sleep. Two years prior, I was hospitalized for an idiopathic bowel obstruction. I began to doubt the wisdom of a 13-hour plane flight, convinced that I would perforate at 35,000 feet. Nonetheless, I made it home without consequence, still with unremitting abdominal pain. After an intense, and thankfully negative, work-up over the next 2 months, I concluded (with my doctors), that I was suffering from separation anxiety!

Although the symptoms abated somewhat, I had decided to accelerate the race to retirement. It is almost as if I had endured the symptoms of separation before the actual event. Now on the other side, I am sure that was indeed the case. Now the symptoms are gone, and I do not miss being tethered to the computer. I do not miss the massive stress of doing complicated (or even simple) surgery. I do not miss the feeling that I never had enough time for things unrelated to work, be it exercise or even mundane tasks around the home. Perhaps this sense of urgency was self-inflicted, but I never learned any other way.

What have I learned in retirement? I learned that retirement is not a loss of relevance, because only the target of relevance changes. Yes, patients benefited from my sense of relevance, but now I want my family and I to be the beneficiaries of whatever relevance I have left. I learned that I do not get back the time I spent working. My father went to work right out of high school, at two blue collar jobs. Without any formal education, he had enough money to support his pedestrian lifestyle for as long as he lasted. He was generous to his children, wait staff, or anyone that provided service to him. He would always tell me "You can't take it with you." It never meant all that much until now. If it were really all about "the money," I should have retired years ago. Yet I learned that it is not easy to escalate one's lifestyle that exceeds one's life-long values. Perhaps I should have paid more attention to my father's advice.

In closing I find myself with a lot of time to reflect, wondering where all the time went. Like my first and last day, I remember the most impactful events, the most difficult patients, the most rewarding cases I have ever done, and the crushing failures. I find myself still worrying about getting ill, putting an abrupt end to my retirement. Fortunately, and surprisingly, the further along I am on the journey of retirement, I am worrying proportionately less. Besides, most things I worry about never happen anyway!

Printed and bound by CPI Group (UK) Ltd, Croydon, CR0 4YY

03/10/2024

01040476-0005